Dear Simon +
Best Wishes!
It was a great
night!

Love
Lisa
♡

lisaB
lifestyle
essentials
get the most out of life

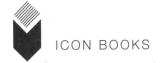

ICON BOOKS

Published in the UK in 2008 by
Icon Books Ltd, The Old Dairy,
Brook Road, Thriplow,
Cambridge SG8 7RG
email: info@iconbooks.co.uk
www.iconbooks.co.uk

Sold in the UK, Europe, South Africa and Asia
by Faber & Faber Ltd, 3 Queen Square,
London WC1N 3AU or their agents

Distributed in the UK, Europe, South Africa and Asia
by TBS Ltd, TBS Distribution Centre, Colchester Road
Frating Green, Colchester CO7 7DW

This edition published in Australia in 2008
by Allen & Unwin Pty Ltd,
PO Box 8500, 83 Alexander Street,
Crows Nest, NSW 2065

Distributed in Canada by
Penguin Books Canada,
90 Eglinton Avenue East, Suite 700,
Toronto, Ontario M4P 2YE

ISBN: 978-1840468-59-5

Designed by Smith & Gilmour Ltd

Printed and bound in Italy by Printer Trento

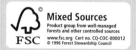

Lisa B is an actress, model, freelance writer and mother of two. Her written work has appeared in a variety of publications including *The Sunday Times' Style* magazine, *Tatler*, *Wedding Day*, and *Pregnancy & Baby*. Her film credits include *Almost Heroes*, *Highlander: Endgame* and *Bridget Jones's Diary*. She has modelled for international magazines such as *Vogue*, *Elle*, *Glamour* and *Cosmopolitan* as well as walking the catwalks for legendary designers such as Chanel, Valentino and Dolce & Gabanna. She recently launched her own clothing range with Crave Maternity and is an ambassador for the International Fund for Animal Welfare, The Brooke and the Dogs Trust, as well as being a patron of Learning for Life and the Foundation for the Relief of Disabled Orphans. She is also the founder of the charitable campaign Mothers4Children.

contents

5 the stylish you

6 the charming you

7 the organised you

8 the balanced you

9 the aspirational you

Throughout the book, you'll see links to the exciting companion website, www.lifestyle-essentials.com. Follow the links to find interactive applications that will help you apply these Lifestyle Essentials to your everyday life.

introduction

Undeniably, we live in a multi-tasking, performance-minded world where there is a growing desire to reassess our lives. No longer is it enough to look good, we need to *feel* good and have organisational skills too. There's immense pressure on us to make the right impression with everything we do while leading such chaotic lives, with little time for luxury, and subsequently we can easily overlook the finer details which can make things that extra bit special. Most importantly, we forget how to conduct ourselves along the way. Almost everyone aspires to having a fulfilling lifestyle, yet many fail to achieve it due to not knowing where to begin.

For me, living is a life's work; there's a foundation to who you are and how you live your life, which constantly needs to evolve, and once recognised, it can attract so much opportunity and possibility. My book explores all the different areas of our lives and attempts to distil the knowledge I've gained, including industry insights from the various worlds I've inhabited, into enriching lifestyle essentials.

I left Brooklyn at seventeen to forge a career for myself and embrace the adventures of life. Although one could consider my beginnings relatively humble, I have always felt great pride, coming from a place that I believe has given me a solid basis to grow from.

Many years of juggling several careers in modelling, film and music (and now being the proud mum of two very young and energetic toddlers!) have enabled me to experience many wonderful things and meet countless remarkable people in England and all over the world, allowing me to lead what many would describe as an 'aspirational' lifestyle.

Through this book, I hope to share some of my insight, help you get the most out of life, and at the very least make you smile and feel good about yourself!

Lisa B

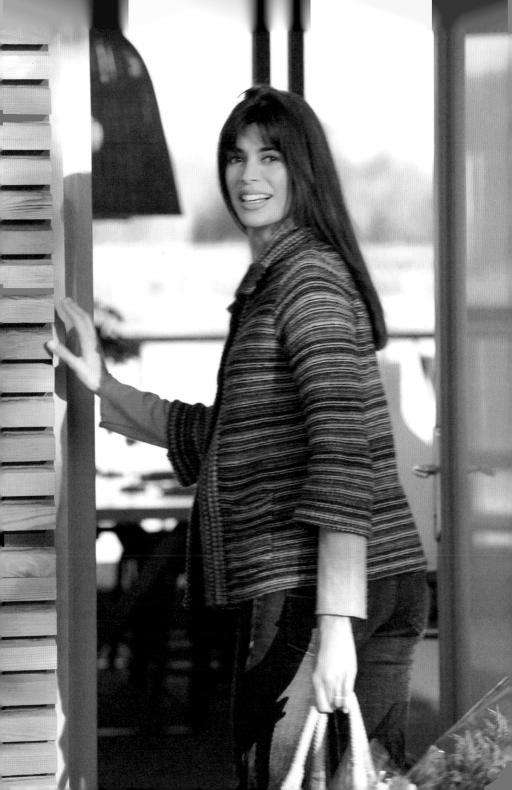

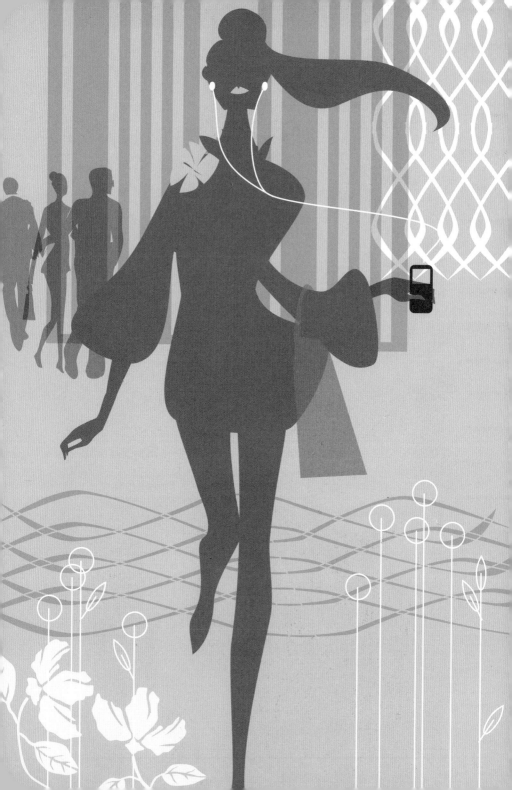

the 1 essential you

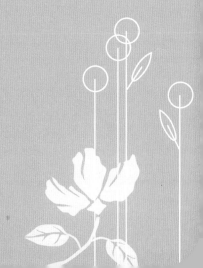

How often do you stop and think about your approach to life? While trying to juggle the many elements of a hectic, modern lifestyle, it's all too easy to accept the way things are and continue on the path that life is mapping out for you. But are you actually making the most of your life?

It's natural to question the way your life is shaping out, especially when experiencing hard times, but it's much more difficult to motivate yourself to make changes. There's no set time or age when you should appraise your lifestyle, so why not step back and take stock today?

There are many elements of yourself that create the bigger picture of how you live your life, and you'll need to look at how you balance all of these different parts. If you identify, assess and develop these parts, you can then build a well-rounded, fulfilled and successful life – but the most important place to start is with your inner self.

'It is your attitude more than your aptitude that will determine your altitude!'
Dr Gary V. Carter

Your inner self

Throughout the course of life you naturally develop your own character, or inner self, as you build relationships with others, cope with difficult situations and participate in different activities. Your sense of self is the fundamental core of you, which affects everything you do and the way you do it. By understanding and strengthening your inner self, you'll be able to develop the different aspects of your life with motivation and enthusiasm.

'Human beings, by changing the inner attitudes of their minds, can change the outer aspects of their lives.'
William James

I like to imagine that living my life is like renovating an ever-changing house – and the foundation of this house is my inner self. Without a solid foundation, the house is more likely to need constant repair and may even collapse completely. In the same way, in order to embrace and overcome life's many challenges, I believe I have to develop strength and confidence from within. The greater this grows, the more anchored and balanced I feel, the more I achieve and the happier I am with my life. Success is measured in many ways, but in my opinion, to be truly successful your achievements should include peace of mind, happiness and great friendships and relationships.

The first question you need to ask yourself is how do you feel on the inside? Be honest with yourself, because who you are and how you feel doesn't only affect your outlook on life, it also affects how others see you. Identify your good attributes and qualities and at the same time look for those you need to develop and nurture. I believe there are many personal attributes that will help you to get the most out of life, including:

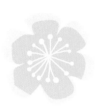

confidence
enthusiasm
forgiveness
humility
integrity
patience
thoughtfulness
tolerance
non-judgementalism
and a good sense of humour!

The positive you

Your sense of self, strength of character and personal attributes affect your ability to cope with situations and ultimately influence what happens to you in life. I firmly believe in 'cause and effect' rather than 'chance'. Good things won't just happen to you – you've got to make them happen. To do this, you need to have a positive outlook. If you always look on the negative side, you'll find that your pessimism prevents you from experiencing new things and achieving new goals.

It's crucial to focus on positive thinking. From this you'll gain confidence, energy, initiative and the will to succeed. The benefits you gain from positive thinking will help you to 'live your best life' – a phrase coined by Oprah Winfrey, which sums it up perfectly. I'm inspired by Oprah's attitude to life – I follow this philosophy myself and think it's something we should all aim to do.

Change your outlook

I consciously make an effort to turn my negative thoughts into positive ones by approaching situations differently. Try reframing your thoughts to help see things in a more positive light – the chart below gets you started on how this is done. It's also a great game to play with the family when in the car, stuck in traffic!

Negative thought	Positive reframe
nosy	enterprising/curious
useless	challenged
disruptive	energetic
complicated	involved
tricky	intricate
obsessive-compulsive	focused
domineering	assertive
vehement	passionate
lazy	indifferent
aggressive	dynamic
angry	aroused
complacent	amiable
nagging	persevering
critical	acute

There's often one major hurdle that prevents us from living our best life and that's fear, or more specifically, the fear of failure – which in essence is negative thinking. It's very important to address this issue when appraising your inner self. It affects our ability to make rational decisions; we become less willing to try new experiences and face new challenges; and it prevents us from moving forward, keeping us stuck in old and familiar routines. Negative thinking can leave us feeling unfulfilled and incomplete, often without even realising why.

It's essential, in your day-to-day life and in setting longer-term goals, that you stop fear holding back the positive you.

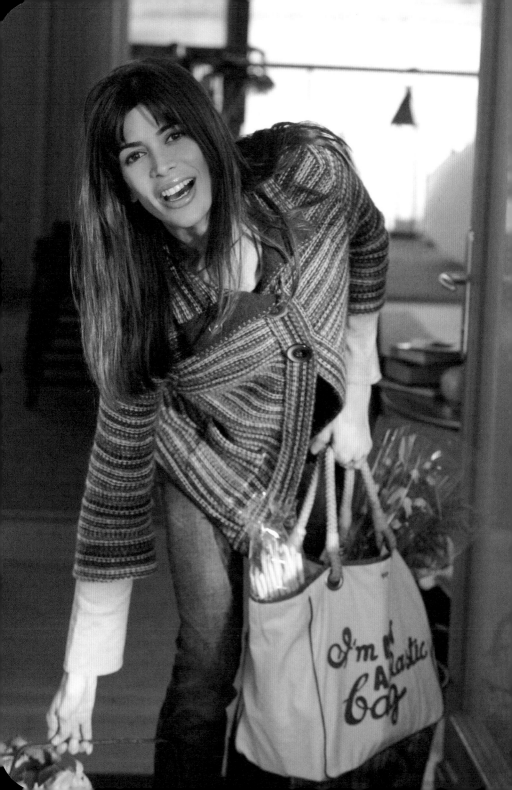

The confident you

There are many steps you can take to help overcome your fears and allow the positive side of you to grow and thrive. Try and focus on the following:

Believe in yourself

Trust your instincts. We all possess a certain amount of innate wisdom; you just need to know how to use it. When you get that feeling in your gut, go with it – it's probably right.

Share your fears

Our fears, no matter how small, can be magnified when we're alone with only our own thoughts. It's often better to share your feelings and worries with a close friend, a member of your family, or even a professional therapist. Another person's point of view can help you acknowledge your fears, keep them in perspective and take positive steps to overcome them.

Positive vibes

Whenever you can, try and associate with people who make you feel good about yourself. It will help you to build a positive self-image and their support and encouragement will give you confidence in your endeavours.

Stay focused

Take time to think about what you want to gain from life. Create a picture of your ideal life in your mind and write down all you hope to achieve. To stay focused on what you want, you need to review this regularly. Don't underestimate the power of positive thought! Every year, I make a new list and keep it on the fridge, where I can see it every day. Yes, a few friends have a chuckle at me, but I always have the last laugh – you'd be amazed how much of it comes to fruition.

Take risks

Let go of attachments that might be holding you back and be prepared to take some risks. Be open to new possibilities and experiences as these are what make life exciting. Embrace change and use it to your advantage.

Set goals

In life we need goals, however big or small, to give us purpose and direction. By setting goals and focusing on attaining them, you learn to use your time more productively and efficiently. You'll enjoy today's tasks much more, knowing they are shaping your future.

Be realistic

Don't expect too much too soon, as this can cause disappointment and a sense of failure. Instead, research what you want to achieve, develop a realistic plan and tackle it in achievable stages. By focusing on what you are able to do right now, you can live in the present – worrying about what 'might' happen is wasted energy.

Stay balanced

Make sure you remember to keep balance in your life, as this is crucial to being happy, healthy and positive. I talk more about how you can do this in **The Balanced You** (p.220).

There seems to be a lot to focus on when trying to stay positive, but always remember – positivity is a state of mind. Be an optimist, not a pessimist and tell yourself: 'Yes, it can be done.'

When I need motivation and inspiration I collect positive affirmations, quotes, poems and words that mean something special to me. When I'm having a bad day, I simply look at my special collection. Give it a try yourself – you'll be amazed at what a difference it can make!

My List of Inspiration

Empowering

'If you can imagine it, you can create it. If you can dream it, you can become it.'
William Arthur Ward

'I would rather fail in a cause that will ultimately triumph than to triumph in a cause that will ultimately fail.'
Woodrow Wilson

'Our greatest glory is not in never falling but in rising every time we fall.'
Confucius

'Destiny is simply having the vision to realize your dreams and the perseverance to keep working towards them.'
C. Phillips

Reassuring

'Life is not measured by the breaths we take but by the moments that take our breath away.'
Anonymous

'Be who you are and say what you feel, because those who mind don't matter and those who matter don't mind.
Dr Suess

Reflective

'An eye for an eye makes the whole world blind.'
Mahatma Gandhi

A journey of a thousand miles starts with a single step.
Anonymous

Humorous

'I know God will not give me anything I can't handle. I just wish he didn't trust me so much!'
Mother Teresa

Poetry

I am only one,
But still I am one.
I cannot do everything,
But still I can do something;
And because I cannot do everything
I will not refuse to do the something
that I can do.

Edward Everett Hale, Lend a Hand

Books

The Alchemist – *Paolo Coelho*

The Road Less Travelled – *M. Scott Peck*

The Seven Spiritual Laws of Success – *Deepak Chopra*

The Celestine Prophecy – *James Redfield*

Songs

1 Spiritual High – *Moodswings feat. Chrissie Hynde*

2 Lean on Me – *Bill Withers*

3 Feeling Good – *Nina Simone*

4 Teardrop – *Massive Attack*

5 We Come One – *Faithless*

6 Rock Steady – *Aretha Franklin*

7 Hang on in There Baby – *Johnny Bristol*

8 Start Me Up – *The Rolling Stones*

9 Beautiful Day – *U2*

10 Respect Yourself – *The Staple Singers*

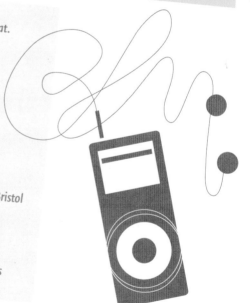

Bring it on!

OK, so now you've taken a good look at your inner self – at who you are and what makes you tick. You've identified the good and bad parts of your personality, know which ones to work on, and how to set yourself goals. You're doing all that you can to stay positive. But, how will this actually affect your life?

To answer this you need to look at all the other areas that make up your life. Use your inner strength and positivity to get the best out of each, so you can be satisfied that you're living your life to the full. With the desire to succeed, and an optimistic and confident outlook, you can set goals in each area and work on achieving them all. Take a look at your health, fitness, appearance, behaviour, family, friends, work and ultimate life goals. Decide what you want for yourself then go out and do it ... there's nothing to stop you now, so bring it on!

'If you can imagine it, you can create it. If you can dream it, you can become it.'
William Arthur Ward

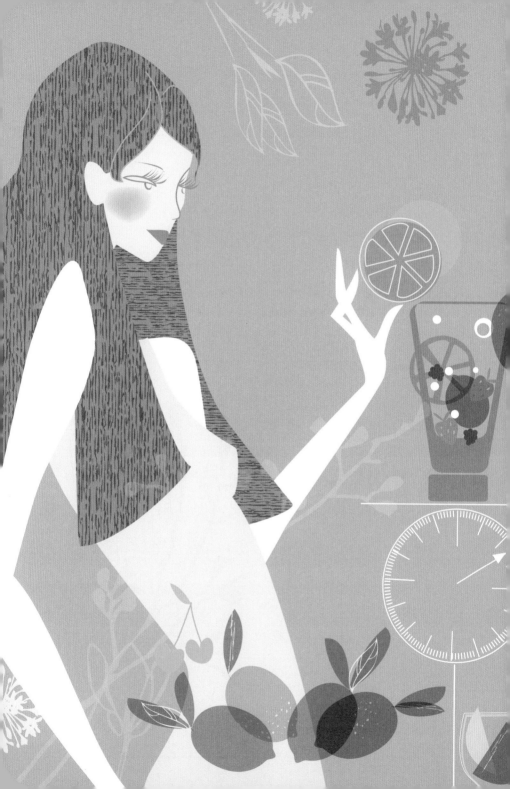

the 2 healthy you

My grandma used to say 'What have you got, if you ain't got your health?' and I couldn't agree with her more. Your health is the most valuable asset you have.

The modern lifestyle we lead inherently affects our health and well-being. Our bodies have to cope with too much convenience food, alcohol, tobacco and stress, and often we don't put enough time aside to look after them properly. As a result, the risk of suffering from certain lifestyle-related diseases – especially heart disease, obesity, depression and diabetes – is increasing.

The best way to help ourselves to stay healthy is to maintain a healthy lifestyle, and to do this you need to pay particular attention to your diet, exercise, stress levels and general health requirements. Take a good look at your lifestyle – what changes do you need to make?

'The greatest wealth is health.'
Virgil

Healthy eating

The phrase 'you are what you eat' is a reminder of the importance of diet and its impact on our health and energy levels. Providing your body with nutritious meals at regular intervals yields many short-term benefits including healthy teeth, skin and hair, a stable and healthy body weight, more energy and an active immune system. In the long term, this also helps reduce the risk of chronic illnesses such as heart disease, strokes, diabetes, cancer and osteoporosis.

Your body needs a well-balanced diet because different food types have different roles to play – and you should eat from the five main food groups every day.

Carbohydrates

(*eg. bread, rice, pasta, noodles, breakfast cereals, potatoes*). As the body's main energy source, carbohydrates should make up 47–50 per cent of your diet. Including at least 18g of fibre a day helps your digestive system work efficiently.

Fruit and vegetables

Try and eat at least five portions a day. Fruit and vegetables are high in fibre, low in calories, and contain a range of vitamins and minerals. It's also believed that they help lower your risk of developing heart disease and some cancers.

Milk and dairy products

(*eg. milk, cheese, yoghurt and fromage frais, but not butter, margarine or cream (all high in fat)*). Various products contain different nutrients but they're all rich in calcium, which strengthens teeth and bones as well as looking after your

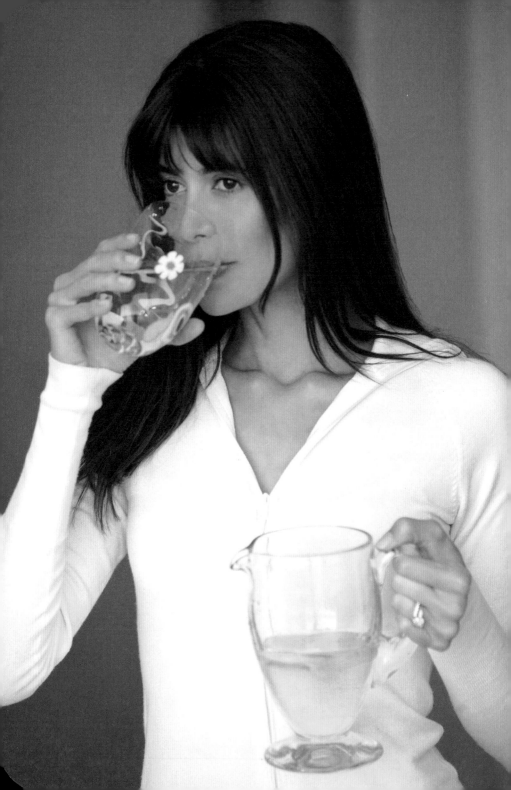

muscles and nerves. To meet your daily calcium needs, you should eat the equivalent of a pint of milk or two pots of yoghurt. You can avoid too much full-fat food by choosing skimmed milk or low-fat cheese and yoghurt.

If you're lactose intolerant, try alternative calcium-rich foods, including green leafy vegetables (like spinach and broccoli), soya milk, rice milk, almonds and dry fruit.

Meat, fish, eggs and alternatives

(alternatives include poultry, Quorn, nuts, seeds, beans, soya products and pulses). These all contain protein, which is the main component of muscle, organs and glands and is crucial for their growth and repair. It's also an important energy provider. However, your body can't store protein so you need a moderate amount every day to replenish levels.

Foods containing fat and sugar

These are a good energy source but contain very few nutrients and lots of calories. Of course they also make food taste better! The good news is that you still need small amounts of them to transport vitamins around your body, cushion organs and even boost your immune system. There are two types of fat – saturated (in butter, margarine, cheese, full-fat milk, etc.) and unsaturated (in sunflower oil, soya, soft margarine and oily fish such as mackerel, sardines and salmon). Unsaturated fat is far healthier, and you should try to minimise the saturated kind in your diet.

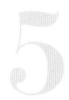

Water

Water's the most abundant nutrient in our body and it's also the most important. It plays an enormous number of roles and is vital

tips

→ Drink a glass of water with every meal and between every meal.
→ Always drink before and after exercise.
→ Dehydration makes a hangover worse, so drink a large glass of water before bed if you've had a few – doubling that with an Alka-Seltzer helps too!
→ Keep a bottle of water in your car in case you're stuck in traffic or travelling long distances.
→ Increase your water intake if you've been sweating or drinking caffeine or alcohol.
→ Every time you go to the kettle to make a cup of tea or coffee, also fill a full glass of water and either drink it before or after your tea or coffee.

for maintaining normal bodily functions, good health and well-being, growth and development. By drinking enough, you also reduce your risk of all kinds of conditions including dehydration, kidney and liver problems, skin complaints, constipation and breast cancer.

It's recommended that you drink around eight glasses (or 2 litres) of water every day to replace the water lost by the body through ordinary activity. Don't rely on tea, coffee and some soft drinks to make up your daily intake, as these are actually diuretics and rather than quench your thirst can leave you feeling thirstier!

Beware the booze

Alcohol affects us all differently but despite its obvious feel-good properties, it can lead to serious illness or addiction if you drink excessively. Studies have shown that alcohol-related death rates in the UK have doubled in the last ten years and are on the rise, with the largest increase in the 35–54-year-old age group. Perhaps it's time to assess your own intake. I enjoy a drink as much as the next person, but remember – all things in moderation!

Excessive drinking impairs judgement and memory, and can make you irrational, angry or depressed. Apart from the most noticeable after-effects of too much alcohol – a blinding hangover can wipe you out for a whole day – it's also worth remembering that alcohol is very high in calories and contains no essential nutrients and vitamins. The serious long-term effects can include:

- addiction
- obesity
- infertility
- muscle disease
- skin complaints
- high blood pressure, leading to stroke
- liver disease
- high cholesterol, and thus heart disease
- some cancers such as mouth and throat
- neurological problems including brain damage and epilepsy
- miscarriage and foetal alcohol syndrome

It's recommended that women drink no more than three units of alcohol a day, with two or three alcohol-free days each week. One unit is generally calculated as 8g of alcohol. To give you an idea of your daily allowance:

1 pint of strong lager = 3 units

1 standard glass of wine (175ml) = 2 units

1 alcopop = 1.5 units.

These recommendations are a general guide, so make sure you're aware of how alcohol affects you personally and set your own limits. Don't be fooled into believing that coffee sobers you up – it's a myth! And if you're the designated driver on a night out, it's probably best to avoid alcohol altogether.

On a more positive note, alcohol is known to have its benefits as well. I find having a glass or two of wine after a long and stressful day relaxes me and can complement a delicious meal. For some, a few drinks help in social settings, allowing them to engage in chat more readily. And it's also been suggested by scientific studies that moderate drinking can also decrease certain cardiovascular disease. Not so bad after all – just remember, moderation is key!

Changing your diet

Now we've looked at the different food groups and why you need them, let's explore food as part of your healthy daily routine.

The fundamentals of gaining or losing weight are not rocket science – they boil down to a simple equation. For weight loss, energy output must be higher than energy input (or vice versa if you're trying to gain weight). Then when you've reached your target weight, you need to change your input and output so they're in balance – the healthiest place to be.

On paper it seems simple, but changing your weight and keeping it stable takes a bit of effort, reasonable discipline and long-term commitment. As I know all too well, the fashion industry's riddled with people looking for a magical pill, cream or the latest miracle diet – most of us are quite lazy and want to shed weight without putting much effort in. Most fad diets focus on one particular food item (anyone for cabbage soup?) or food type (low-carb, low-fat, high-protein). But the truth is, the majority of these leave out essential nutrients and vitamins and keep your weight yo-yoing – both of which can lead to serious health problems now and in the future.

If you want to make long-term changes to your weight, then avoid fad diets and other 'quick-fix' solutions. Instead focus on a healthy lifestyle, which means eating well and exercising regularly to burn energy and build muscle, fitness and strength.

'When it comes to eating right and exercising, there is no "I'll start tomorrow."'

V.L. Allineare

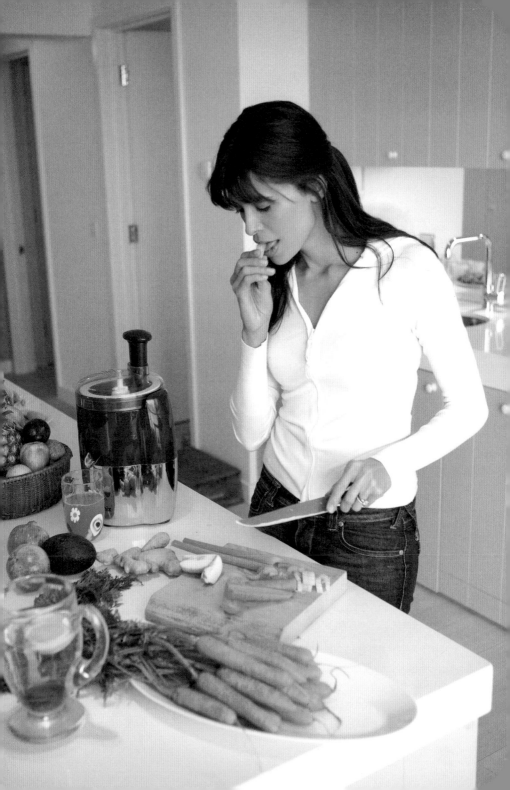

Four steps to a healthy diet

Avoid very restrictive diets

Anything that dramatically limits your calorie intake is neither sustainable nor healthy – it deprives your body of the nutrition it needs. You might lose a lot of weight in the short term, but it's not worth battling with low energy, poor concentration, food preoccupations, constipation, terrible mood swings and irritability. Plus your metabolism will slow down as you go into starvation mode – your body will hoard every last calorie, meaning when you finally come to your senses and quit the diet, you'll pile the weight on. Need I say more?

Adopt healthy eating habits

Enjoy a balanced diet: make sure you eat lots of fresh fruits and vegetables, lean proteins, fish, pulses, beans and unprocessed carbohydrates. Start eating healthily today and make it a long-term goal to keep doing so. Adopt the attitude that you're treating yourself by eating well, and not depriving yourself. I can guarantee you'll feel better for it!

Start slowly

Remember – Rome wasn't built in a day. If you've been used to eating poorly or too much, you need to give yourself time to adjust. Trying to change your eating habits too quickly might mean you give up and slip back into old habits.

Keep a food journal or diary

Keeping an accurate overview of all the foods you consume on a daily basis will clearly show what you are eating and if you are lacking balance within your diet. Seeing things written down is often hugely helpful. Record every morsel that passes your lips – also include the quantities. If eating is an issue in terms of binging or not eating enough, record the time you ate throughout the day, where you ate, how you felt before and after you ate, so you can begin to recognise how your emotions affect your eating.

Quick food tips

- It's better to snack between moderate-sized meals than to have three large meals each day. Just make sure they're the right snacks – keep a stock of healthy treats on hand – dried or fresh fruit, veggie sticks, nuts, rice cakes, etc.

- Poach, steam or grill food instead of frying.

- Don't skip breakfast! A healthy breakfast refuels your body and jumpstarts your day. I usually have two slices of toast with peanut butter, or two eggs – either boiled or scrambled. During winter, I love a bowl of porridge with a sprinkle of brown sugar. Yum!

- Don't starve yourself. Your body needs fuel, and without it you'll just be hungrier throughout the day and end up eating more. Try to eat at least three meals a day.

- Eat in proportion to your exercise levels – if you do a heavy workout then you need to eat more than if you've been resting or inactive.

- Try not to comfort eat. Avoid fast foods as they tend to be prepared in oils made of saturated fats.

- When eating out, conjure up a healthy meal plan beforehand and try to stick to it. Look for fish, white meat and steamed vegetable options but stay away from fried, heavy or creamy foods.

- Eat a light snack, such as an apple, an hour before exercising.

Lisa's meal plan

Breakfast   Multi-grain toast with peanut butter, a banana, fresh carrot juice from the juicer, cup of tea

Lunch   Soy, lemon and honey marinated chicken breast grilled on a green leafy salad with sliced avocado, an apple

Snack   Cadbury fruit-and-nut chocolate bar, cup of tea

Dinner   Baked salmon with a honey and mustard glaze and chopped cherry tomatoes, steamed asparagus with lemon and oil dressing and shaved almonds, side dish of basmati rice with caramelised onions

* Glass of water with each meal and several throughout the day

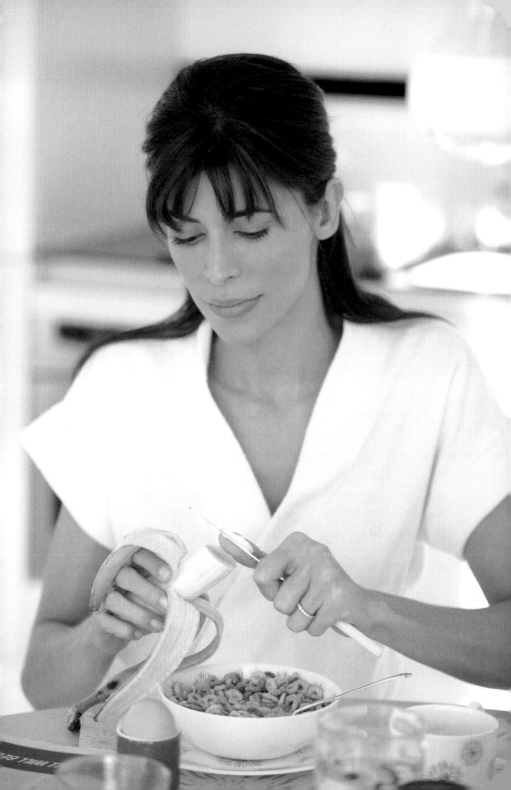

An ideal weight

Women's weight has been a pretty controversial topic of late, especially with all the recent attention on the new size zero.

Being a model, I've always been extra aware of my weight. It's definitely difficult to feel totally balanced about your weight when it's always been under a microscope.

There's also a lot of criticism of the fashion industry for its negative influence on women – which adds another dimension of pressure. While some days I feel like I'm carrying a little extra weight, most days I feel I'm a little too thin – I've got one of those annoyingly fast metabolisms where I burn off calories faster than most, and have to eat more just to keep the weight on.

I'd never want or intentionally influence girls to be underweight, but as a model, it could easily be suggested that I do. But rather than place blame on individuals, I think it'd be far more beneficial for the fashion and celebrity industries to promote girls of all different shapes and sizes – as long as they're healthy! It's also important to remember that many images of already slim models and celebrities are retouched and don't reflect reality at all – further distorting women's perceptions of what is an ideal body weight.

Since having my children, I've achieved a balanced weight that I'm happy with. I make sure I'm never too busy to eat properly – I need to be strong, healthy and full of energy to keep up with the two of them!

'So what is a healthy or ideal weight?'

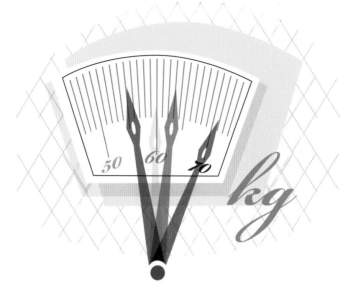

Body Mass Index

A combination of factors determines each person's weight – we all have different frames and body shapes – and that's why it's difficult to set a single measure that applies to everyone. The good news is there's a healthy weight range we can use as a guide – and you can check if you're within it by using the Body Mass Index (BMI), a calculation based on your weight and height.

formula:

$$BMI = \frac{weight\ (kg)}{height\ (m) \times height\ (m)}$$

example:

$$BMI = \frac{60\ kg}{1.65\ m \times 1.65\ m} = 22$$

BMI ranges

Underweight	→	less than 18.5
Ideal	→	18.5–25
Overweight	→	25–30
Obese	→	30–40

'It's important to make an objective yet accurate assessment of your size – it's easy to under- or overestimate your own weight.'

Be aware that your idea of what makes an 'ideal' body weight might not actually be a healthy one. Being outside the normal range can lead to serious health problems, so if you need to gain or lose weight, ask your GP for advice, and look at what lifestyle changes you can make.

Medical history

It's very important to make sure you know your own body. On a general level, you should know your own basic medical details and history – vaccinations, appointments, advice, procedures, treatments and medication. On a more personal level, you should be aware of your body and look for changes that may cause future health problems.

Often, when I need my medical information and details of previous treatments, I actually can't remember, which is very frustrating. Your doctor will have records but if you're away from home, or in an emergency, you really need to know yourself. To ensure that I'm always aware of the basics I've created my own medical history folder. You can download my template from www.lifestyle-essentials.com – or create your own using the guidelines opposite.

my medical history

NAME: *Lisa B*

DATE OF BIRTH:

BLOOD TYPE:

KNOWN MEDICAL CONDITIONS:

CURRENT MEDICATION:

DRUG ALLERGIES:

GENERAL ALLERGIES:

FAMILY HISTORY:

DOCTOR'S DETAILS:

IMMUNISATION RECORD:

TREATMENT/OPERATIONS:

HEALTH INSURANCE POLICY DETAILS:

NATIONAL INSURANCE NUMBER:

→ **Doctor (GP)**
→ **Nearest emergency surgery**
→ **Dentist**
→ **Optometrist**
→ **Gynaecologist**
→ **Dermatologist**
→ **Chiropractor**
→ **Nearest pharmacy**
→ **Specialists**

It's also very useful to create a list of medical contacts to save you having to flick through address books in the event of an emergency. I've done this for myself and my family and keep copies in easily accessible places – near the phone, in my diary and on my computer. They include the name, address, contact details and any relevant notes for each contact.

If you have a young family, keep track of each family member's medical history as well, using the same template.

Health checks

It's vital to have regular medical checks to give yourself peace of mind that you're in good health and doing all you can to stay that way. We consider it totally normal to take our cars in for a regular service, so it seems crazy that many of us fail to do the same for ourselves. Think of what a complex system the human body is, and of the daily wear and tear we put it through!

It's common for people, especially those under 40, to think that they don't need to visit a doctor. But even if you feel fine now, you should be aware of any measures you can take to prevent, as much as possible, serious illness developing in the future. Where your health is concerned, prevention is definitely better than cure. Regular check-ups can also help catch potential health problems early, increasing the chance of successful treatment.

There are several suggested screenings and checks that women should have on a regular basis, and depending on your medical history and the medical history of your family, there may be some you need earlier or more frequently than recommended. It's best to play it safe and if you have any concerns or need professional advice, don't hesitate to consult your GP.

'An ounce of prevention is worth a pound of cure.'
Henry de Bracton

Self-awareness checks

It's very important to be aware of your own body and to recognise any changes. Whatever your age, there are some basic health checks you can do yourself.

Vaccinations

Check they are up to date, including any additional requirements, such as a flu jab. This is easily kept on top of by keeping a vaccination record.

Weight

It's healthiest to maintain a stable weight and make sure you're not too over- or underweight. For more information, see **An ideal weight** on p.34.

Breast examination

As any doctor will tell you, the most effective way to fight breast cancer is to detect it early, and so it's crucial to familiarise yourself with the shape of your breasts and watch out for any changes or abnormalities. Try and make a regular self-examination, say once a month, to check your breasts for lumps or thickening of the skin. It's recommended that you make your checks three days after your period. I find it easiest to check my breasts while in the shower or lying in bed (you should actually check both standing and lying down).

If you haven't checked before, try the steps on the following page.

You can download my template at www.lifestyle-essentials.com

Before you get into the shower, inspect your breasts in front of the mirror, with your arms at your sides; with your hands on your hips; and then with your arms raised above your head. Look for changes in contour, appearance of the nipple, swelling or dimpling of skin.

Once you've had a good look at your breasts, you can do the rest of your check while standing in the shower – it's easier when your hands are wet and soapy. Using your fingers, press firmly on your breast, checking the entire breast and armpit area. Move around both your breasts in a circular, up-and-down, or wedge pattern (moving fingers towards the nipple).

Check your nipples for discharge (fluid), by gently squeezing the tissue surrounding the nipple and pulling outward.

Also examine both breasts lying down. To examine the right breast, place a pillow under your right shoulder and place your right hand behind your head. Using the pads of your fingers, press firmly, checking the entire breast and armpit area, then repeat for the left breast.

Ask a doctor ...

Remember, at all times, if you have any type of health problem or physical symptom, DO NOT self-diagnose or self-medicate, but speak to a medical professional.

Sexual health

I doubt anyone reading this book needs any insight on the 'birds and the bees', but you'd be surprised about how many myths there are when it comes to sexual health. Unfortunately, too many sexually active people have forgotten or are ignoring the need for safe sex. Sexually transmitted diseases (also known as STDs) are on the rise, so it's imperative to be responsible for your own sexual health.

High-risk STDs

Chlamydia – The UK's most common STD, this is a bacterial infection which can affect the cervix, genitals, urethra, rectum and sometimes throat or eyes. Most people show no symptoms, although indications can include discharge from the vagina or penis, or pain when urinating.

If left untreated, it can spread to other parts of the body and cause health problems such as reduced fertility or infertility.

HIV (Human Immunodeficiency Virus) and AIDS – HIV/AIDS is the most dangerous of the STDs. It's now more common in heterosexuals than homosexuals, and can infect anybody regardless of age, sex, ethnicity or sexual orientation. All penetrative sexual acts carry a risk of infection, but always using condoms can reduce this risk.

Gonorrhea – Also known as the clap, this bacterial infection infects the genitals, rectum, urethra and throat. There's a small chance of having no symptoms, but most people infected notice

facts

→ There are three ways to transmit sexually transmitted diseases: through vaginal, anal and oral sex.

→ Always use condoms during sex, unless both partners are certain that they do not have an STD.

→ Be aware that condoms can protect against some STDs but not all. Some infections like genital warts and herpes, among others, can still be transmitted.

→ Not all STDs have obvious symptoms so get tested if you've been careless or forgetful.

→ The pill does not protect against STDs.

unusual discharge from the penis or vagina and pain when urinating. If not treated, it can spread to reproductive organs, causing reduced fertility and possibly infertility.

Genital warts – Genital warts are caused by some types of Human Papilloma Virus (HPV) and are passed on through penetrative sex – direct skin-to-skin contact. They appear singly or in groups as small lumps on the genital area, although they may be invisible. Other symptoms include burning or itching. It's best to be checked for these by a nurse or doctor, as there can also be hidden ones internally. Although they don't generally cause any long-term health problems, they can develop into more serious infections or indicate the presence of more dangerous HPVs which may be associated with changes in cervical cells that can lead to cancer. Women can be checked for this during a cervical smear test. Genital warts are treated with swabbing, freezing, laser treatment or surgery.

Genital herpes – There are two types of herpes: one which affects the mouth and the other, the genitals. Herpes is contracted through direct skin-to-skin contact during sex, including oral sex, or even by kissing. The symptoms can include a tingling in the genital area, which is then followed by blisters leading to painful sores. Sadly, once contracted, there's no treatment to successfully rid your body of the virus. It comes and goes periodically and pills help clear up outbreaks as they occur.

If you have any concerns, ask your GP for an STD check or visit a sexual health clinic.

Contraception

Contraception is mainly used to prevent pregnancy, although condoms also protect against some STDs. The most common forms of contraception besides condoms are the pill (the hormones of these are also available as injections or implants now), physical barriers such as cervical caps or diaphragms, or an IUD (intra-uterine device) which is placed in the womb by your doctor. Everyone reacts differently to the various forms of contraception, especially the hormonal methods (pills), so it's best to discuss options with your GP to find the birth control best suited to you. When making recommendations, your doctor will consider your sexual lifestyle, age and medical history. Contraception is provided free on the NHS, so ask your nurse or GP for more information.

The morning-after pill

Also known as the emergency contraceptive, the morning-after pill is used the day after having unprotected sex to stop you from becoming pregnant. It can actually work for up to three days after sex and is about 90 per cent effective, but the earlier you take it the better. The controversy about the pill stems from not understanding what it does – it's not an abortion-causing drug and it won't actually work if you are already pregnant. Your GP can prescribe it, or you can now buy it over the counter from your local pharmacist.

Regular medical checks

Health screens are designed to look for evidence of disease in people showing no symptoms of the particular illness. Detection at an early stage will increase the likelihood of successful treatment. Over the page is a list of the most important checks, showing at what age and how frequently they should be carried out.

For more useful medical info, reminders and checklists, visit www. lifestyle-essentials.com

Cervical screening

Between the ages of 20 and 65 it's important to have regular smear tests to detect early cell abnormalities that, if left untreated, could lead to cancer of the cervix. The cervix refers to the lower part of the womb, or uterus, and cancer of the cervix is the sixth most common cancer in women in the UK. The tests are free and you will be invited to have an initial test before the age of 25. From 25–49 years you should have a test every three years; from 50–64 you should have a test every five years and from 65+ you will only need further tests if you've recently shown abnormalities.

Many women receive a result showing borderline changes, which usually return to normal without any treatment. If this happened to you, you'd be asked to return for an extra test in six to twelve months' time to check that cells are healthy, and then generally return to the routine checks.

New vaccines have recently been developed for Human Papilloma Viruses (HPVs), which are the major cause of cervical cancer, but these are not yet available within the UK.

Blood pressure

High blood pressure increases the risk of developing serious conditions such as heart disease and stroke. The higher your blood pressure, the higher the risk. Blood pressure can change over time so it's important to be tested every 3–5 years.

Cholesterol

Your body has a natural supply of cholesterol, but too much in the blood can increase the risk of cardiovascular disease such as angina, heart disease and stroke. You're more at risk if you're overweight or diabetic, if you eat too much saturated fat, smoke or don't exercise enough. The ideal level is 4–5 and you should have an initial check around the age of 30 to find out if you need to make any lifestyle or dietary changes to keep it stable. If there's a history of heart attacks in your family you should get tested regularly.

Blood sugar
Blood sugar tests check the amount of glucose (sugar) in your blood. If levels are above the safe range then you may be suffering from diabetes, which can be monitored and kept in check. After the age of 40 you should have your blood sugar levels tested every five years, especially if you're overweight.

Eye test
If you have never had an eye test, make an appointment with an optician to do so as soon as possible, especially if your work involves lots of close-up reading or working on a computer. There are various eye conditions that don't immediately impact on your vision. An eye test only takes around 30 minutes. Your eyesight changes over time, so try and have a check-up every two years. This is especially important once you hit 40, because the risk of eye diseases such as glaucoma increases.

Extra checks for women over 50
As you get older, you become more at risk from certain conditions. It's important that you're aware of the following checks to look after yourself and your body.

Breast screening – In the UK a free screening service for breast cancer is offered every three years to all women between 50 and 70. You should continue to check your own breasts as well.

Osteoporosis – After the age of 60, it's recommended that you have a bone density scan to detect any weakness or vulnerability that would increase the risk of breaks and fractures.

Bowel cancer – Screening is recommended every two years for anyone aged between 50 and 69.

Men's health

Men often do all they can to avoid visiting the doctor, so the men in your life – whether your partner, husband, brother or father – might need a few reminders and a nudge in the right direction! Funnily enough, it was actually my health-savvy husband who made me realise that, while you don't need to be obsessive about it, it's incredibly important to be aware of your own health and also that of your partner and family.

These days I'm aware of both female and male health risks and what to be watching out for. A great friend of mine was diagnosed with testicular cancer a few years ago – and was only in his mid-twenties, which was a real wake-up call to me. Just because you're young, it doesn't make you immortal.

Many of the things men need to do are just the same – monitoring any changes in their body, having up-to-date vaccinations, keeping a check on weight, BMI and sexual health, along with all the recommended checks for blood pressure, cholesterol, blood sugar and eyesight.

But these following checks are specific to men – and it's helpful to understand yourself what is involved.

Testicular cancer

This is the single biggest cause of cancer-related deaths in men between fifteen and 35. Symptoms include a lump in one testicle, pain or tenderness, discharge or pus, a build-up of fluid inside the scrotum, a heavy feeling in the groin, an increase in testicle size. There's a high success rate for curing this disease, especially if diagnosed early, so it's important to check for abnormalities regularly, and visit a doctor immediately if any develop. Lumps or changes are often due to a less serious condition, but need to be checked.

Prostate problems

Prostate cancer is the most common cancer in men, especially those over 60. Symptoms include difficulty or pain in urinating, needing to do so more frequently, or feeling like the bladder hasn't emptied properly. Any changes in urinary patterns, particularly in men over 40, should be checked straight away with a doctor – many common problems can be treated and kept under control. Other symptoms of prostate cancer include lower back pain, pain in the hips or pelvis, blood in the urine, difficulty in getting or keeping an erection. Men over 50 should have a prostate test every two years, even if they're not showing any symptoms.

For more detailed information and links, head to my website – www. lifestyle-essentials.com

Colorectal cancer

Colorectal cancer, or cancer of the bowel, is the third most common cancer in men. It's found predominantly in men over the age of 45. Men with diabetes or with a family history of bowel cancer could be more at risk. Symptoms include blood or mucus when emptying bowels, a lump in the abdomen, diarrhoea or constipation lasting more than two weeks, stomach pain or discomfort, weight loss and fatigue. These symptoms could also be due to other bowel problems but should be checked out by a GP.

First aid

Does your household have a first aid kit at the ready? It's always best to be prepared, as you never know when somebody might have an accident or get sick. Here's a list of medical supplies that it's sensible to keep on hand – make sure you keep a check on the use-by dates of all the medicines.

essentials

→ Absorbent dressing
→ Antacid
→ Antihistamine cream and tablets
→ Antiseptic – wipes or liquid
→ Assortment of plasters
→ Cold/flu medicine
→ Cough syrup
→ Eye pads
→ Eye wash solution
→ Ibuprofen/aspirin
→ Petroleum jelly
→ Gaviscon
→ Safety pins
→ Scissors
→ Tape
→ Thermometer
→ Throat lozenges
→ Tubular bandage
→ Tweezers
→ Vinyl gloves

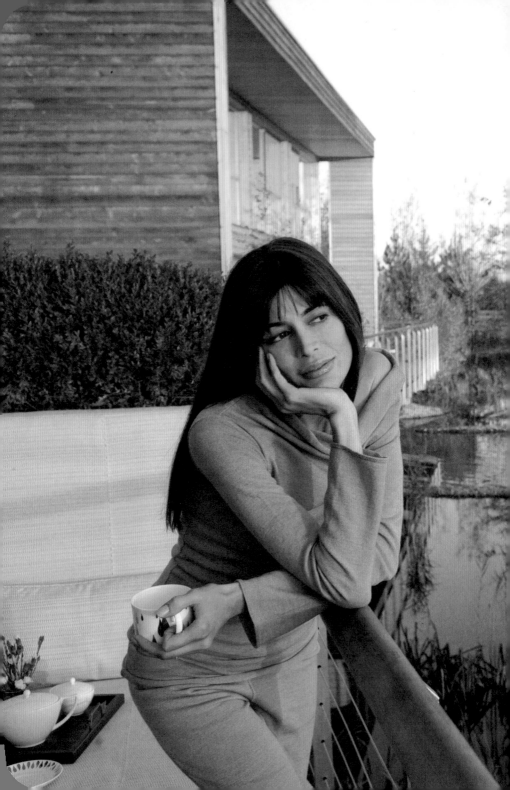

Stress

Ginger and lemon tea

This is great for a bedtime drink, a relaxing spa evening in, or if you're beginning to feel a little under the weather.

1 Add sliced fresh ginger to the biggest mug you can find (start with small slices to test strengths)

2 Add one slice of lemon and a teaspoon of organic honey

3 Pour in boiling water and let steep for several minutes

Fresh mint tea

You can serve this after dinner as an alternative to coffee. It's great for digestion as well. I also enjoy drinking it before I go to bed on cold winter nights.

1 Place a handful of mint leaves into a teapot, pour over boiling water and let steep for several minutes

2 Drink as is, or with a small amount of organic honey

Stress-related medical problems are becoming increasingly common as we learn to deal with the difficulties and challenges of modern life. Stress is the tension you feel when there are too many demands on you – and we all have different ways of dealing with it. You may find stress acts as a stimulant, driving you on, or you may find it depresses and demotivates you. Most of us can cope with short periods of stress but being exposed to long periods can cause emotional and psychological disruption as well as affecting our physical health.

Symptoms vary greatly between each individual but things to look out for include: irritability or anger, depression, anxiety, concentration problems, loss of appetite, comfort eating, tiredness or sleeping problems, skin problems, tight back and neck muscles, low sex drive, and tension headaches. In extreme cases of stress you may shake, hyperventilate, sweat and feel nauseous.

In order to minimise your stress, you need to identify the aspects of your life that cause stress and work out how to counteract them (if, for instance, you're under a lot of pressure at work, you could set out a plan to prioritise and balance your workload and voice your concerns to your manager). The important thing is to take action sooner rather than later and make changes. I talk more about keeping a low-stress lifestyle in **The Balanced You** (see p. 220).

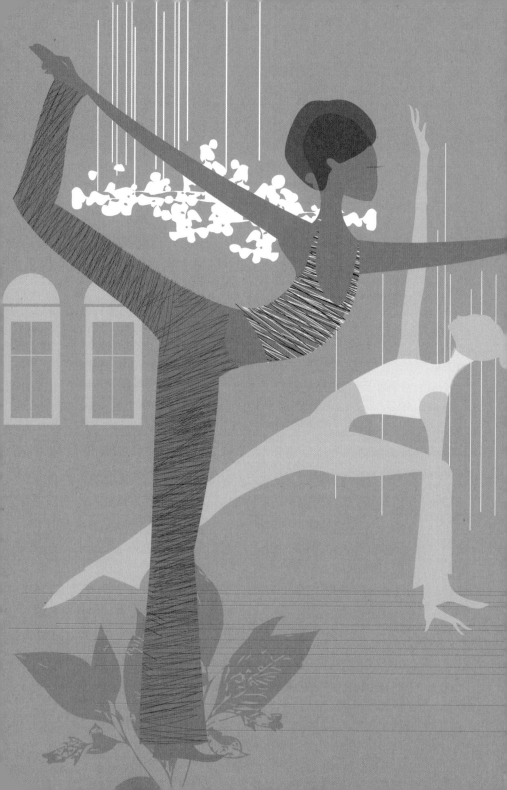

the 3
fit you

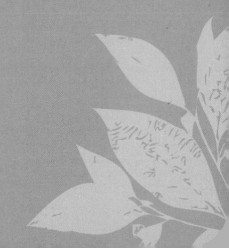

Wouldn't it be great if we could just take a 'fitness' pill – one which kept our figures trim and toned and allowed us to eat as many puddings as we wanted to? Lovely thought though it is, that's all it will ever be. The key to getting and staying fit is the good old-fashioned balance between exercise and good nutrition – with the two of these you'll be well on your way to a healthy lifestyle. We've already looked at the benefits of healthy eating in the last chapter, and now we'll look at how exercise improves the way you feel, inside and out.

Modern life means that many of us don't engage in physical activity in our everyday routines. Without making a conscious effort to exercise, it's all too easy to travel to work, sit at a desk all day, come home and then, after you've finished the chores, park yourself in front of the TV for the night. The pressures of family life can make it difficult to set aside enough time for exercise. There are also some women who feel self-conscious about their body and sporting ability, and so avoid group exercise.

However, when you understand the benefits of regular exercise, you'll see that it's essential to make your fitness a priority and find an exercise programme suitable for you.

'Fitness – if it came in a bottle, everybody would have a great body.' Cher

The benefits of regular exercise

Only 24 per cent of women in the UK exercise enough to really get any benefit from it. At a minimum, adults should do 30 minutes of moderate physical exercise five days a week (the 30 minutes can be spread throughout the day rather than in one go). And recent studies are recommending that to reap the full health benefits, more vigorous activity is needed.

Exercise helps you live a longer and happier life, and has positive influences on other parts of your life as well. Chemicals known as endorphins are released into your brain during exercise – these lift your mood, make you feel good and also combat stress. Also, exercise is an opportunity to help you meet new people, discover new interests and generally feel better about yourself.

Improved fitness has many benefits, but here are eight of the most important:

1 General health

Exercise improves your digestion, posture, circulation and blood pressure.

2 Healthy heart

Coronary heart disease generally results from the build-up of a fatty deposit inside the lining of the arteries, which causes them to narrow and increases the risk of angina and heart attack. Lack of physical activity is one of the highest risk factors for heart disease; exercising regularly lowers your blood pressure, reduces cholesterol, improves circulation and decreases the likelihood of fatty build-up on your arteries.

Stable weight

Exercise, along with a balanced diet, helps you maintain a stable weight, or lose weight if you need to. In addition to all the health benefits, this makes you feel happier about your appearance and boosts your self-confidence.

Strong bones

All exercise helps strengthen muscles, joints and bones. In particular, weight-bearing exercise, such as running or aerobics, helps promote bone density and reduces the risk of osteoporosis later in life.

High energy

Although exercise can be tiring at the time, it does in fact boost your energy levels in general. As you become fitter, your body learns to cope with more, so once you establish your exercise routine you'll feel less tired.

Mental health

The feel-good effects and increased self-confidence given by exercise aid good mental health, help manage stress and anxiety, and even prevent depression. Working towards exercise goals can also give a sense of achievement and pride and increase self-esteem.

Better balance

Certain types of exercise improve your balance, coordination, mobility and suppleness (you'll reap the benefits of this when you get older).

Improved sleep

8

Most people find they sleep better after exercise, although exercising late at night can give you an endorphin high which might not wear off by the time you go to bed. If this is the case, time your workout in advance of bedtime!

Getting started

The key to exercise is finding a form and level that suits you. We're all individuals who will benefit from and be naturally drawn to different types of exercise. It's crucial that you find a form of exercise that you find fun – there's nothing harder than forcing yourself into a gruelling workout, dreading it beforehand and hating every minute. You can tell yourself, 'no pain, no gain', but ultimately you need to find an activity that appeals to you if you want to stay motivated and focused.

When setting your exercise plan, it's also important to look at your current health and lifestyle and consider the key elements of fitness.

- Cardio-respiratory exercises – work your heart and lungs
- Muscular endurance and strength exercises – rely on your ability to hold specific positions or repeat movements (with or without weights)
- Flexibility exercises – rely on your ability to move joints and muscles through a full range of motions

The most effective regime will combine these elements and address your fitness strengths and weaknesses.

If you don't already exercise regularly, maybe all you need is a little motivation, encouragement and enthusiasm. To get geared up and focused on getting fit, decide on an exercise plan that works best for you.

When it comes to my fitness plan I'm not a creature of habit – and need a variety of activities to stay interested. I've always been someone who goes to the gym for workouts – because I enjoy taking different classes. I find music hugely motivating, so I go for classes like salsa, modern jazz, or hip-hop/stress-dance classes, or even some power yoga classes – all of which are driven by funky upbeat music, inspiring a great workout. I try to incorporate the free weights and machine workouts for toning and strength and also occasionally work with a trainer for certain periods (I did this after both of my pregnancies). I find this really keeps me fit – along with walking everywhere I can, and running after two young children and a very energetic husband!

Whether you go to a gym, use a personal trainer, prefer a group class, try a team sport, exercise alone or fit it into your everyday routines, there is truly something for everyone, leaving no excuse for not being as fit as can be!

In the gym

If you think you'd benefit from constant motivation or social contact then an ideal environment for you is a gym. It's a great place to work on your overall fitness and muscle strength. Look for one that's clean, with up-to-date equipment as well as friendly and helpful staff, and check the selection of classes they have on offer. Make it easier and less time-consuming to exercise by finding a gym near your work or home.

Gyms usually offer a range of cardiovascular machines (like treadmills, cross-trainers and static bikes), resistance equipment for weight training (machines and free weights) and a wide variety of fitness classes, such as aerobics. Some gyms may also have additional facilities such as swimming pools and squash courts.

Unfortunately gyms can also be very expensive. You usually have to pay a monthly or annual membership, but this entitles you to unlimited access to all facilities. It might be worth checking if your gym offers special packages or off-peak rates if they suit your routine, and also check the minimum membership period in case you decide it's not for you after all. Before signing up for full membership, check for any introductory deals, such as initially paying for casual sessions or joining for a trial period of time, to make sure you're happy with the gym.

Paying in advance can make you determined to get your money's worth, meaning you'll be less inclined to skip sessions and more likely to continue with your exercise programme. But there are also many council-run fitness and leisure centres throughout the country which allow you to pay per session. You still have to pay for your induction and possibly a small joining fee, but the benefits are usually worth it!

When you join a gym, a qualified instructor will usually assess your health and fitness levels, as well as giving you an induction to the various machines and weights. You should also be given advice on technique to prevent injury and a training programme based on your individual needs so you can then train by yourself.

To keep motivated you might want to book sessions with a personal trainer, which are often well worth the money. Make sure the trainer is qualified to recognised standards. Alternatively, try organising a training partner or 'gym buddy' to work out with you – maybe a friend, partner or someone you've met at the gym. By spurring each other on, you might find you progress much faster!

Group classes

As I've already mentioned, classes are without a doubt my favourite way to keep fit – especially the ones which incorporate dance and great music. Play a bit of Beyoncé and Destiny's Child and I'm happy to 'shake my thang' for hours! There are numerous fitness classes available at all levels. Group classes can be more sociable and fun than gym workouts, especially if you're the type of person who can't get motivated alone. It often takes a few sessions to build up your confidence and understand how the routines work in a class – so stick it out if you find the first one difficult!

Classes will vary from gentle, non-impact types to highly energetic fat-burning options. To give you an idea of the variety available, here's a list of the most popular classes.

Low-impact and toning classes

Yoga – Yoga is believed to be one of the most effective, relaxing and gentle forms of exercise, not only for the body, but also for the mind. Most traditional styles of yoga have three basic principles in common: controlled, focused breathing; performing a series of postures or poses; and meditation to focus the mind and relax the body.

Pilates – Pilates is a popular mind–body conditioning exercise. It aims to promote neuromuscular harmony, balance and coordination, while increasing strength and flexibility. Each movement is executed according to six basic principles: control, concentration, centring, focus, precision and breathing. Pilates is something new I've recently tried to help strengthen my lower back. After two babies, it's now the weakest part of my body, and I want to prevent this from becoming more of an issue as I age.

Aquarobics – This cardiovascular and conditioning class takes place in a swimming pool and uses the water resistance to strengthen and tone, with minimum impact on joints. It may be done in shallow or deep water (deep water being harder).

Abs and Butts – A shorter version of the above, focusing on buttocks and abdominals.

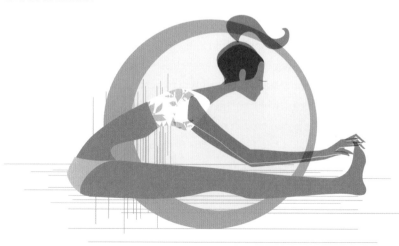

Legs, Bums and Tums – Suitable for all levels, this toning class focuses on thighs, buttocks and abdominals – great for helping to reduce cellulite!

Fat-burning workouts

Aerobics – Aerobics is done to music and can be highly choreographed. Classes are designed to burn fat and improve fitness, stamina, coordination and flexibility. A range of aerobics classes are available, including Hi/Lo (where you pick your own level) and Step (working on and off a plastic box).

Kick Boxing/Boxercise – Includes boxing techniques. Body Combat is a martial-arts-based workout, and Dance Aerobics incorporates high levels of choreography and dance routines.

Spinning – This is a workout to music using static bicycles where you can vary the resistance and speed of the pedals depending on your level and ability. A high-energy calorie killer, it's also good for joints as it only involves minimum impact.

Body and muscle conditioning using weight resistance

Body Pump – This offers a range of exercises using barbells with adjustable weights and is set to music. It works all major muscle groups of the body.

Circuit Training – A combination of cardiovascular and resistance work performed at various stations each for a set duration. Focusing on repetition, this is an excellent way to improve strength, stamina and flexibility.

tips

→ Check out a class first to make sure it's right for you

→ Speak to the instructor if you're not sure what's involved

→ Wear comfortable clothing – start with a T-shirt and shorts or tracksuit, and if you like the class, invest in specialist clothing

→ Wear trainers with non-marking soles

→ Take water with you, ideally in a plastic bottle

→ Take a towel

→ Tell the instructor if it's your first time, or if you have any injuries or medical problems

→ Don't eat a meal for at least an hour before a class

→ Don't expect to perfect all the moves immediately – everyone was a beginner once!

Team sports

Team sports are not only fantastic for getting fit, they're an automatic way of meeting a whole load of new people, and the feeling of team spirit can be hugely rewarding. If you're not ultra-competitive, consider joining a social league – you can form a team with your friends, or ask the organisers if they can place you on a team. Having a fixed time to exercise can be a great way of making sure you show up – especially when you know others are depending on you.

Go it solo

You might prefer to work out outside of a gym and save the cost of membership or regular class fees. There are many activities you can do at flexible times that don't need expensive equipment or any expertise.

Running

The good thing about running is that you can do it almost anywhere and it's a very effective way of getting fit. All you need is a good pair of running shoes. However, running is a high-impact activity and can put stress on your joints. You should check with your GP before running if you've ever experienced chest pain, asthma, epilepsy or high blood pressure.

Swimming

Most towns have a swimming pool and you don't need much sports gear to get going! It's a great way to tone up using the resistance of the water, with no impact on your joints. Swimming works most major muscles and is also an effective fat-burning method, especially if you can build up the distance. If you can already swim, try improver lessons to perfect your technique.

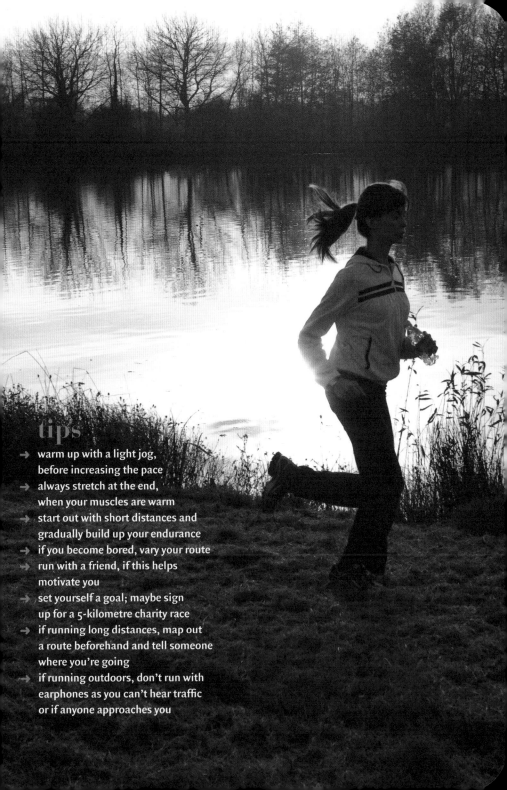

tips

→ warm up with a light jog,
  before increasing the pace
→ always stretch at the end,
  when your muscles are warm
→ start out with short distances and
  gradually build up your endurance
→ if you become bored, vary your route
→ run with a friend, if this helps
  motivate you
→ set yourself a goal; maybe sign
  up for a 5-kilometre charity race
→ if running long distances, map out
  a route beforehand and tell someone
  where you're going
→ if running outdoors, don't run with
  earphones as you can't hear traffic
  or if anyone approaches you

Cycling

Many people own bikes but don't actually use them. As long as your bike is safe and reliable and you have a good helmet there's nothing to stop you enjoying a quick spin! I've got a brilliant bike, which has a pod-like attachment at the front, so both my little ones can sit in it as I cycle along – it's a great way for us all to enjoy some fresh air. Cycling provides a cardiovascular workout and because the bike supports your body there is minimal impact on your joints. It's also a good way to burn fat – about 300 calories per hour. Enjoy a leisurely cycle ride in the country or use your bike for any short trip that you'd usually do in your car or by tube. You'll be surprised how good it makes you feel!

Dancing

Who doesn't like to dance? Everyone has some form of music which inspires or motivates them to move, and that's all dance is – coordinated movements. Dancing is an aerobic activity but doesn't really feel like it – with a great tune playing, it almost feels effortless. Dancing builds your fitness, stamina and flexibility, while giving you a chance to make new friends. Don't be put off by thinking you don't have any coordination. Find a beginners' class and give it a try – I guarantee everyone else will be just as nervous as you! Classes are run all over the place – school halls, village centres, sports centres and even church halls – and there are countless types of dance to try.

Walking

This is probably the easiest form of exercise to do and costs nothing at all. It's good for your heart, lungs and leg muscles and you can use it to get you to where you need to be, or choose a path with enjoyable scenery. Walking increases your oxygen intake, which helps burn calories, and is less likely to cause injury than other types of exercise.

Home gym

Having a gym at home is incredibly convenient – no need to drive, find parking or wait for machines. But before you go off and spend big bucks on cumbersome and expensive equipment, try working to a regular routine at home for a month or two first (for instance, running round a block and using a skipping rope and free weights). If you stick to the plan, then the gym equipment may well be a worthwhile investment. But if you lose interest, then don't waste your money. I speak from experience – my husband bought a rowing machine, which he only ever used once, and it now sits like an art installation in our laundry room!

Top fitness tips

- Choose a programme that suits your personality and your lifestyle.
- If you're new to exercise, begin your routine slowly and incorporate small amounts at a time. Include a variety of cardio and flexibility exercises and avoid heavy weights until you've been shown how to use them properly.
- Get a friend or partner involved. Getting fit together helps encourage you and stops you from getting bored. It's good for their health too!
- Set realistic goals. You'll feel boosted with achievement whenever you reach them.
- Always include a warm-up and muscle stretches in your exercise routine. Stretching improves flexibility and reduces the risk of injury and soreness.
- Work up to your maximum potential slowly and stay focused. Increase activity levels progressively so your body adapts before being asked to do more.
- Always pay attention to your body. If you feel weak or tired, don't force a workout as you will be less productive.
- For any health concerns or injuries resulting from exercise, always seek medical advice straight away.

Exercise alternatives

I think I can speak for a lot of people when I say it's possible to have a real love/hate relationship with exercise. Personally, some days I love it and some days I really hate it! When I was pregnant, I definitely hated going to the gym, so followed a workout DVD at home to keep myself motivated and active.

Maybe you think that going to the gym just isn't for you. Or maybe your life is just too busy to fit in a regulated exercise programme and stick to it properly. Don't worry! Just remember – anything is better than nothing, so try adapting your current lifestyle to fit your activity needs.

If you want to be a bit more organised about it, create some kind of training plan so you still have some kind of fitness goals to work to, and hang it on your fridge where you can easily see it. You could add in new goals for each week and check them off when done. Make it more fun by rewarding your achievements – just not with chocolate cake, or anything fattening!

You can think of ideas that will suit you personally but here are a few to get you started. It isn't cheating … it's still exercising – honest!

tips

→ Clean your house for 30 minutes – burn up to 135 calories
→ Wash your car for 25 minutes – burn up to 100 calories
→ Garden for 30 minutes – burn up to 100 calories
→ Use the stairs instead of taking the lift or escalator
→ Walk short trips instead of taking the car, taxi or bus
→ Walk briskly between shops and use that shopping trip to burn calories
→ Carry shopping bags to get taut, toned arms
→ Walk or cycle to work
→ Work your neck muscles, shoulders and back with simple exercises at your desk
→ If sitting in one place for long periods of time, move your legs or flex and point your feet – or grip a book between your knees to strengthen your thighs
→ Do abdominal crunches, push-ups, or leg lifts while lying on the floor watching TV
→ Walk or march in place while watching television
→ Dance around the living room to your favourite music
→ Get a fitness DVD and work it into your weekly schedule at home

Get the gear

Keeping fit is good for your health but let's be honest – we also pursue fitness because we want it to make our bodies look good. With this in mind, it's important to choose workout gear that helps you look good, as this in turn can add incentive to keep up with your training programme. After all, if we look good, we feel good.

Workout clothing

When considering what to wear to the gym, it's important to choose clothing that you feel confident in, so you don't feel too self-conscious. The good news is, sportswear has come a long way and companies like Nike, Puma and Adidas now create incredibly stylish workout clothing that suits women of all shapes and sizes. I have to say, shopping in the giant Nike store in New York was enough to motivate me into a desire to up my fitness. Even fashion designers have started incorporating sportswear into their collections – check out Stella McCartney and DKNY for outfits that even the most fanatical fashionista would be happy to work up a sweat in.

Most importantly, sportswear should be comfortable, allowing you to move, bend and stretch easily. Your workout gear should breathe as well as offering some form of support. Where possible, choose clothing with a mix of cotton and synthetic materials such as spandex, polyester, nylon or acrylic. Sports clothing is designed for specific types of workout but what generally looks and feels best is a fitted T-shirt or tank top with gym trousers, tracksuit pants or shorts (not bike-shorts!).

Good workout clothes aren't cheap, but are worth the investment. If you can, go out to a fitness clothing store and treat yourself – kit yourself out from head to toe in something you really like and feel good in! Think of it as a reward for keeping fit.

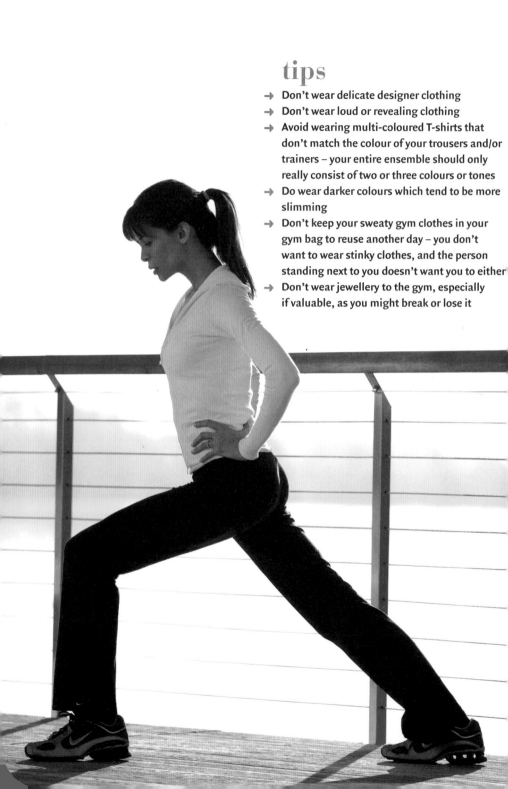

tips

→ Don't wear delicate designer clothing
→ Don't wear loud or revealing clothing
→ Avoid wearing multi-coloured T-shirts that don't match the colour of your trousers and/or trainers – your entire ensemble should only really consist of two or three colours or tones
→ Do wear darker colours which tend to be more slimming
→ Don't keep your sweaty gym clothes in your gym bag to reuse another day – you don't want to wear stinky clothes, and the person standing next to you doesn't want you to either
→ Don't wear jewellery to the gym, especially if valuable, as you might break or lose it

Sports bras

Are a must! When working out, it's crucial that your breasts are supported, restricting excessive movement. Choose a material that breathes, yet is very supportive – one with Lycra is ideal. Try on a variety of different sports bras to find the right one for you. It should fit snugly without cutting into the body and should also be easy to move about in. Try jumping about, running on the spot and also stretching to make sure it fits well and gives the support you need.

Footwear

There are lots of different types of training shoes so it's important to choose those that best suit your workout. Any good sports shop should be able to help you if you explain what you'll be using them for. Remember to take along the same type of sock you work out in, and also try on a good selection until you find the pair that feels just right. Before you buy them, test them out properly, by walking and jogging around the store and jumping up and down.

Trainer types

Cross-trainers – These are the most commonly worn trainers because they're versatile and can be used for a whole range of workout activities – walking, running, gym training or fitness classes. They offer stability and durability and tend to be wide at the bottom to allow easier side-to-side movement. Make sure they offer good support, are flexible and well cushioned.

Running shoes – If you plan on doing lots of running then it's better to buy a specialist running shoe rather than a cross-trainer as they're designed specifically for the forward-and-back stride motion. Generally running shoes are a size or a size and a half larger than your normal footwear, and you should leave a thumb's width (or half an inch) between your longest toe and the end of the shoe. A running shoe should hold your foot securely around the arch, instep and heel.

Walking shoes – Designed specifically for walking, these are generally very comfortable and offer cushioning, motion control and support. If you'll be mainly walking off-road, on rural tracks, you may find trail shoes better adapted to the terrain.

Socks

Always wear socks with your trainers when working out! Choose socks that allow your feet to breathe and for high-impact classes look for socks with padded toes and heels for extra protection from blisters. The most common sports socks are white or grey and made from a blend of cotton and synthetic material. Don't wear dress socks with trainers!

Gym bag essentials

There are several items you should consider stocking up on, depending on how much exercise you do and what your gym already provides.

- Start by finding a bag big enough to carry everything you need – avoid leather bags, as you may need to carry wet and sweaty clothing inside it.
- If the lockers at your gym don't already have locks attached, take your own lock to keep your valuables safe.
- You never know when you may need a little extra energy, either before or after a workout, so keep some healthy snacks in your bag. Energy bars (granola bars are good) or a bag full of almonds are ideal.
- I find listening to my favourite tunes on my MP3 player very inspiring and motivating when I work out. You could create a workout playlist with upbeat music for the workout and then more relaxing tunes for cooling down and stretching. You need to decide the best way to carry your player – maybe clipping it onto a belt or arm band.

- You need water to rehydrate – and lots of it! There are great water bottles you can buy specifically for working out, with an attachment to drink from so you don't need to stop what you're doing or spill water all over yourself.

- Using weights, especially free weights and bars, can cause calluses and blisters on your hands so if you plan on lifting weights, invest in a pair of weight-training gloves, to prevent this happening.

- If your gym doesn't provide towels, take one to wipe away sweat or lie on during your workout, and one for use in the shower.

- Wear flip-flops in the changing room and showers to prevent catching any foot infections.

- Depending on what toiletries your gym provides, pack all that you need – essential lotions and creams, shampoo and conditioner, body wash, make-up, deodorant, tampons etc.

- Remember your hairbrush, hair ties, clips and hairdryer (if there isn't already one at your gym). Keep your hair tied back and off your face while working out – it will only annoy you.

- With items like toiletries, hairbrushes, hair bands and so on, I buy two sets and leave one set at home and the other in my gym bag so I'm not constantly filling or emptying my gym bag every day. Otherwise it's too easy to forget something essential!

- Having a training worksheet to log your daily routine and exercise levels can help keep you motivated. You can download a template from www.lifestyle-essentials.com.

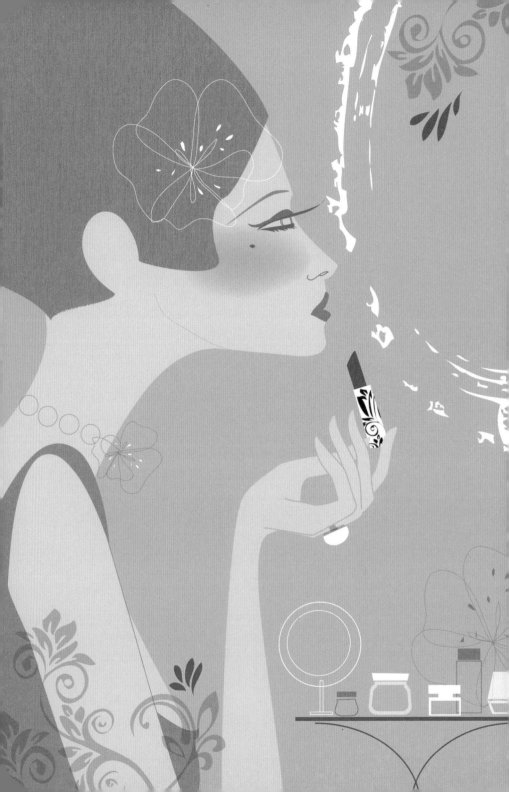

the 4 beautiful you

We've already talked about how to look at your inner self to identify strengths, work on positivity, and provide yourself with a stable base from which to build. The self-confidence you develop on the inside will become invaluable when shifting your attention to your outer self – your appearance.

Attention to outer beauty has been very relevant to my life – both as a model and from working in the entertainment industry for over eighteen years. If there's one thing I've gained from my time modelling – it's definitely thick skin! The biggest irony about models is that – despite public perception of them as 'the beautiful people' – more often than not, they tend to be the most insecure people you'll ever meet. Part of the reason, I believe, is that they become the focus of constant attention, with unrelenting pressure to always look good. The tender age of most models doesn't help – so many people lack confidence when they're young, even without all the extra scrutiny.

True beauty

Confidence, or lack of it, can greatly affect how women, including models, see themselves on the outside. It's all too easy to feel doubtful and insecure about our looks, given the continual images of 'beautiful people' shown in the media. The 'Hollywood ideal' can warp your perspective on reality, causing you to place expectations on yourself that you feel you'll never attain. But trust me – having been in the business for over eighteen years now, I can verify that the world of entertainment is made up of illusion, with a lot of delusion on top of that!

We're all individuals with different qualities. You need to remember that you're unique – and use this to your advantage. Remember, also, that a terrible personality overshadows any purely external beauty. I've known many a self-obsessed model who on a magazine page were gorgeous beyond belief, but having met them in person, I could no longer see their beauty. It's often confidence, with the right balance of humility and a great personality that makes a person strikingly attractive to others.

The first step towards recognising and making the most of your own beauty is working on your self-image. The way you see yourself also affects the way others see and treat you. Believe in yourself – you need to make sure you have a positive attitude towards yourself and like the personality that you project. It might be useful to make a list of the things you like about yourself and things you think others like about you. I'm sure you will be pleasantly surprised!

'The absence of flaw in beauty is itself a flaw.'
Havelock Ellis

Your self-image

Your image is not only how others form their first impression of you – more importantly, it affects the way you feel about yourself and the way you act. The good news is you have control over your image, and every now and again you should put in a little extra effort to make any changes you think will be beneficial. Sometimes it's scary to make these changes. Many people fancy a new hairstyle or new fashion look but aren't sure if it will suit them, so they stick with what's safe instead. But how will you know if you don't try new things? Otherwise, you're going to be stuck with the same hair you've had for the last ten years!

Start by giving yourself an assessment or image overhaul. It might help identify areas you want to change, and your good points that you want to keep or enhance. You should consider the following points.

Personal appearance

Your appearance is a good starting point for evaluation. We're often judged by the first impression we make so it's important to take a look at what others actually see. This includes your total look and sense of style from head to toe – your wardrobe, make-up, hair and so on. By making a change, however slight, to your everyday appearance, you can inject a whole new sense of energy and confidence into your life.

● Analyse your wardrobe – does it need an update?
● Do you wear colours and styles that suit you and your shape?
● Have you had the same hairstyle for years? Try a new one.
● Are your teeth healthy? A nice smile can make all the difference.

Body language

Body language makes up at least half of our communication with the outer world – as the saying goes, 'actions speak louder than words'. How we carry ourselves sends messages and emotional cues just as clearly as what we say. Consider what your body language says about you in various situations. Work towards being more open, thoughtful and graceful with your body language.

- Consider how you sit, stand and generally move
- Be aware of your posture – hold yourself confidently and stand tall
- Consider how you look at people – try and maintain eye contact, smile and keep a pleasant expression
- Do others regard you as approachable or do you appear aloof and uninterested?

Communication and attitude

Your attitude can change the way others see you and behave towards you. You can look as good as you want, but if you have a bad attitude, you will find you get treated less favourably. A negative or poor attitude might not be intentional so take a close look at yours. Getting on with, listening to and enjoying others is a very important part of life.

- Address your general manners; are you thoughtful and kind? See chapter six for a closer look at manners and how to behave.
- What tone of voice do you use? Do you come across as aggressive or dismissive? Maybe you appear to be timid and meek.
- Take a genuine interest in others by listening to what they have to say and focusing on the things you know they are passionate about. Ask questions and show a willingness to learn more about them.

You will need to work on your own body language and communication skills to assess and change whatever you need to improve the way others see you. With your appearance, however, there are more general things you can do and more guides I can give to help get you started.

The graceful you – ageing with style

A woman who defines 'ageing gracefully' to me is Audrey Hepburn – no matter her age, she always was the embodiment of elegance and grace. She's still often voted at the top of lists of natural beauties – and while it's not known whether she ever had any work done, if she did (a big if in my opinion), it was certainly extremely subtle.

I doubt Audrey Hepburn had any extraordinary secrets to remaining youthful and I wish I could say that in my eighteen years of modelling I've found the magical Fountain of Youth, or miracle cream or pill. But I'm afraid that the only wrinkle-free guarantee is the airbrush tool on Photoshop!

Basically, there are two choices when it comes to the inevitable process of getting older: you can be miserable about it and fight it every step of the way – which I believe will only help you age more quickly – or you can embrace it as part of life's journey.

Now don't get me wrong – I don't mean you should accept the stereotypes of age. I'm all for looking and feeling as young as possible. But ageing gracefully is a matter of self-esteem. The key is to feel happy with ourselves every step of the way – our lines, our scars, our years – these are all part of who we are ... The question: What are the four signs of ageing?

'They are wisdom, confidence, character and strength – look for them not with dismay, but with hope.' Valerie Monroe

Age with grace

- Accept that change is inevitable and don't fear it – don't get hung up on numbers such as age, height or weight.
- Enjoy the wisdom that comes with age.
- Take care of your health and well-being and enjoy a healthy lifestyle – stay active and interested in life.
- Stop and enjoy the simple things in life that really give us pleasure – joy and pleasure are what keep us young! Living and enjoying life help keep you young.
- There's a great saying that really rings true to me –'Be alive, while you are alive.'

Age with style

- Take care of your skin – moisturise your face, wear suncream and don't lie in the sun.
- Consider a new haircut – it can really take years off! Ask your hairdresser for some youthful ideas.
- If considering cosmetic surgery, start with non-invasive or non-surgical procedures first, such as facial massages and laser treatments. Anything you are considering injecting into your face should definitely be non-permanent!
- Dress your age – this doesn't mean be dowdy and conservative, but strive for a certain style and elegance.
- Keep your wardrobe up to date – add and subtract pieces each year to modernise your look.
- Ultimately – how you dress should make you feel and look good and say something positive about where you are at in your life.

The beauty basics

Thanks to years of modelling, I've tried and tested just about every beauty tip, secret and product you can imagine, but I have learnt one fundamental lesson – keep it simple. You can spend endless money on cosmetics, skin products and treatments to look younger, smoother, firmer and healthier – but most of it will be in vain. It's much more beneficial to simply concentrate on taking care of yourself. Take my grandma as an example. She's over 90 but doesn't look a day over 70. Aside from probably having good genes, she has cleansed and moisturised her face every morning and evening using an inexpensive cocoa butter formula, has never been greatly exposed to the sun and has never smoked.

Following a basic skincare routine will encourage great-looking skin. Combine this with a healthy diet and lifestyle and you'll see the benefits of a youthful and natural beauty.

Skincare

Adopt the steps below in your daily routine.

Cleanse

Always cleanse your face daily. In the morning I use a gentle foaming wash and in the evening a gentle cleansing wipe and a splash of water. I choose brands which say 'Gentle' or 'For sensitive skin' as they will be less likely to dry out my skin. Use an alcohol-free toner to deep-cleanse your pores. It's often said that you shouldn't squeeze spots but personally I disagree. Any build-up within your pores should be removed or your pores will stretch, becoming big and unsightly and hard to get rid of.

To unclog pores, try placing a hot towel over your face for a minute or two in the evening, then gently work the skin around the pore with your fingertips. Take great care when squeezing – you might want to use a tissue over your nails so you don't damage the surface of your skin. It's best to do this before bed so your skin has time to recover. Once you've cleared the pores, splash some cool water over your face and pat dry. If any are difficult to clear, leave them for the time being and try using a facial mask the next day – picking too much and too hard will damage the skin. If you've got troublesome acne or blemishes, try products containing salicylic acid, glycolic acid, chlorhexidine, benzoyl peroxide, or more natural products containing tea tree oil.

Moisturise

Moisturising is essential to keep your skin soft and supple and protect the cells. Choose a moisturiser to suit your skin type – oily, dry or combination. I have to admit that although my grandma uses one faithful moisturiser and looks amazing, I tend to use two different ones – one for day and one for night. You may also need more than one moisturiser if your skin has especially dry and oily patches. And your daytime moisturiser should include a sun protection factor (SPF) of 15–30+.

In the daytime, I use a light, oil-free one for my entire face. I let it sink into the skin for a few minutes before applying any make-up. At night, I use a heavier cream-based moisturiser and some vitamin E oil on the dry patches and under my eyes. Don't forget to moisturise and use an SPF on your neck! Make-up and good skincare may hide your age but a neglected neck will betray you!

Sun protection

The sun's rays – ultraviolet A (UVA) and ultraviolet B (UVB) are damaging to your skin. Your face is at particular risk from harmful rays as it's the most exposed part of the body. Continual exposure to the sun can cause dryness, fine lines, wrinkles and skin cancer, so avoid direct sunlight on your face whenever possible. A bit of colour on your face may give a 'healthy glow', but be aware of the dangers – too much sun is far from healthy! Wear a high protection factor sun cream and be especially careful if you have naturally fair skin, freckles, moles or a history of skin cancer in your family. Remember – the sun's rays are strongest between 11 am and 3 pm and can even reach you through cloud cover, so your best bet is to stay in the shade or keep a hat on.

Smoking

Aside from the obvious long-term health risks associated with smoking, it's also bad for your skin. Toxins released into the blood supply cause collagen levels to deplete, making the skin thinner. This affects the face in particular and can accelerate the normal ageing process. As a result, smokers will often display signs of premature ageing – such as an increased number of fine lines and wrinkles, particularly around the mouth – and their skin may also have a general grey appearance.

Drink lots of water

Keeping yourself hydrated promotes good skin growth and reduces the occurrence of skin complaints. See my helpful water tips on p.26.

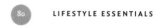

Facials

Facials are a wonderful way to keep your complexion glowing and gorgeous; not only are they beneficial to your skin, they can also be very relaxing. Because of my busy schedule, I often find it easier to give myself one at home than to visit a professional (although that's always a lovely treat). I love using a wonderful mask by Aveda called Tourmaline Charged Radiance Masque. Try your own home facial, following the steps below.

1 Tie your hair back from your face.

2 Cleanse your face of any make-up.

3 After you've cleansed, apply a facial exfoliant to remove dead skin. Use circular and upward motions, but don't rub too hard, before washing with clear warm water.

4 Fill a large bowl with boiling water from the kettle and drop in a few drops of your favourite essential oil. One of my favourites is ylang ylang – its scent is floral, exotic and uplifting and helps enhance your relaxation.

5 Hold your face over the bowl and cover your head with a towel to keep the steam aimed at your face (this will open your pores and soften your skin).

6 Choose a mask to suit your skin type. After you've applied it, rinse or peel it off after the suggested time. Use cool water to rinse your face thoroughly, and then pat dry.

7 Apply a toner using a cotton-wool pad – this helps close your pores.

8 Finally, apply a moisturiser to nourish and protect your skin.

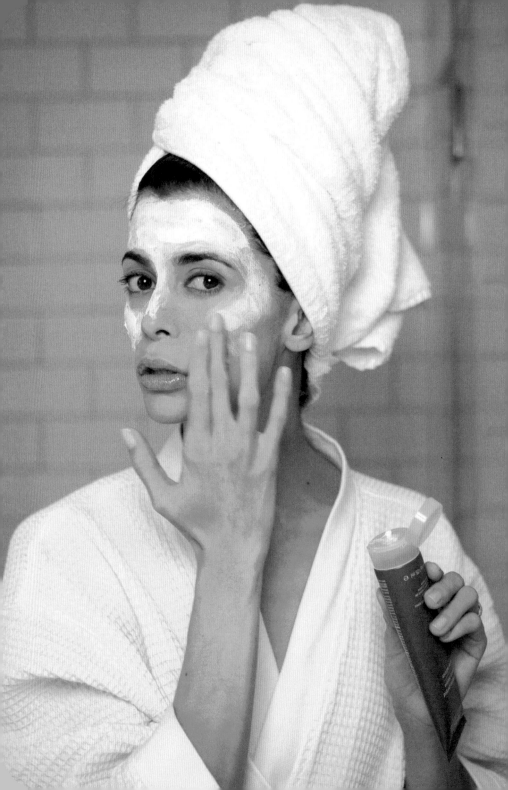

Make-up

Media portrayals of beauty seem to focus on unattainable perfection, which many women then aspire to. What you need to remember is that make-up used on models and actresses in front of a camera is applied by a professional artist and isn't the same as the make-up you use from day to day. Furthermore, we too often forget what's commonly known – how often the modelling and entertainment world uses the art of retouching. It's one of the biggest tricks of the trade and practically every one of those perfect, blemish- and wrinkle-free faces you see these days in magazines, newspapers and even music videos has probably been retouched. Thanks to retouching, I could probably model until I was about 80 without a care in the world if I wanted to!

Here in the real world we don't have the luxury of a personal make-up artist or the ability to retouch our image, so we need to learn a few tricks for ourselves. It's important to understand that make-up is actually very individual. Some girls can't leave home without it; some can't bear wearing any at all. Some colours look amazing on certain skin tones, yet make others look dreadful.

Even with the vast amount of make-up products on the market, it can be difficult to find the right ones for you. There are several factors you should consider when choosing and applying make-up – your face shape and skin tone, your look and style, and even your mood. Make-up is about changing, empowering and even playing!

Applying your make-up

Learning how to apply make-up properly takes a bit of practice and a lot of trial and error! On a day-to-day basis I personally prefer to wear what looks most natural, as I think a little can go a long way. On big nights out it's fun to be a bit bolder, so I wear stronger make-up to define my features more, but I still lean on the side of caution when applying my 'look'.

These two basic types of make-up – daytime and evening – both call for different shades and techniques. However, it's important to remember that – whether for day or night – the purpose of cosmetics is to enhance a woman's natural beauty, by minimising skin imperfections and accentuating facial features.

One thing you should know before you invest in a variety of make-up types and colours is what type of complexion you have. Basically, skin tones fall into two categories, warm and cool, and are classified as dark, olive or yellow, rosy, tanned, or fair. Try holding a piece of white paper up to your face and identify the main colour you see. This should help you identify your skin tone.

Another hugely important tip is to apply your make-up in a well-lit area. In the morning, I apply my make-up near a window, so I can see what it will look like in natural daylight. When using artificial light, make sure it hits your entire face evenly, not just from above, as you don't want any shadows. Just to be safe, I check my face in several lights before I go out!

Follow these steps to apply your base make-up perfectly ...

Moisturiser

Apply your moisturiser a few minutes before you apply anything else, especially if you have dry skin and spend a lot of time outside. Let it sink into the skin. Choose a moisturiser with an SPF (at least 15+) to protect your skin from harmful UV rays. If you have great skin and don't need much coverage, use a tinted moisturiser and skip using a foundation but make sure the tinted moisturiser blends evenly into the skin.

Concealer

Choose a concealer one shade lighter than your actual skin tone and blend evenly over blemishes, minor imperfections, dark circles under the eyes etc. You can use a cosmetic sponge for this, although I prefer to just use my fingertips. Only apply small amounts at a time because too much concealer can exaggerate or create lines on the face, which might cause a 'cakey' or 'raccoon-like' effect around the eyes.

Foundation

If there's one item of make-up you should not skimp on it's foundation, so try and buy the best you can afford, as the variety of tones available are so much truer to real skin tones. Foundations generally have either a golden- or blue-toned base, with variations that flatter a wide group of faces in the warm and cool ranges. Basically, if you have cool skin, choose a foundation that has blue or pink undertones, and use a yellow-base foundation for warm skin. Foundation comes in liquid, stick or moist-powder form and should be used sparingly to even out the skin tone. This will give the appearance of smooth, blemish-free skin.

Stick foundations tend to give you more coverage. I love Bobby Brown's foundation sticks, which I apply with my fingers. I have a lighter shade for winter and another slightly darker shade for summer – then I can also blend the two together to perfectly match my skin tone whatever the time of year. The moist-powder type foundations offer a two-in-one combination of both foundation and powder – they are quick and easy to apply and great for keeping in your handbag for retouches. My favourite is Mac's Studio Fix. Again I have two shades and blend the two to get more natural coverage. Powder-based foundations are generally better for oily skin, while liquid foundations give less coverage but can be oil-free, and are best applied with a moist cosmetic sponge.

Choose a foundation as close to your skin tone as possible. You shouldn't see the make-up on your face – if you do, you're using the wrong shade.

Powder

Finishing powder is optional and is applied after your foundation has been absorbed, to help it set. Once you are happy that the concealer and foundation are blended well and look as natural as possible, dust a translucent powder lightly over your entire face with a large applicator brush. If there's any colour in your powder, it should be as close to that of your foundation as possible.

Blush

Blush gives your cheeks colour, contour and a healthy glow. It usually comes in a pressed powder form, which should be applied with a blush brush, or as a cream, which can be applied using your fingers. If using a cream, apply it before your powder.

When choosing a blush, pay special attention to your skin tone. It should also be about two shades darker than your foundation. For a daytime look, choose soft colours, but for going out at night you can choose darker, shimmery colours, which add more highlight to the cheek.

Select a colour that will suit your skin tone

- **Fair skin tones** – pink, tawny and beige
- **Olive to yellow skin tones** – copper, almond, and warm browns
- **Tanned skin** – peach, coral, apricot and orange
- **Darker skin tones** – plums, auburns and rich bronzes

Eyebrows

Some eyebrows need filling in and shaping, which can be done with an actual eyebrow pencil or by applying eye shadow with a very small brush. If you have dark eyebrows, use a colour a shade lighter than your hair colour so they don't end up looking too dark. Only fill in sparse areas and blend if necessary.

Once your base make-up has been applied, you can then consider the look and colours you want for the rest of your face – depending on whether it's for day or night and according to how much make-up you wish to use ...

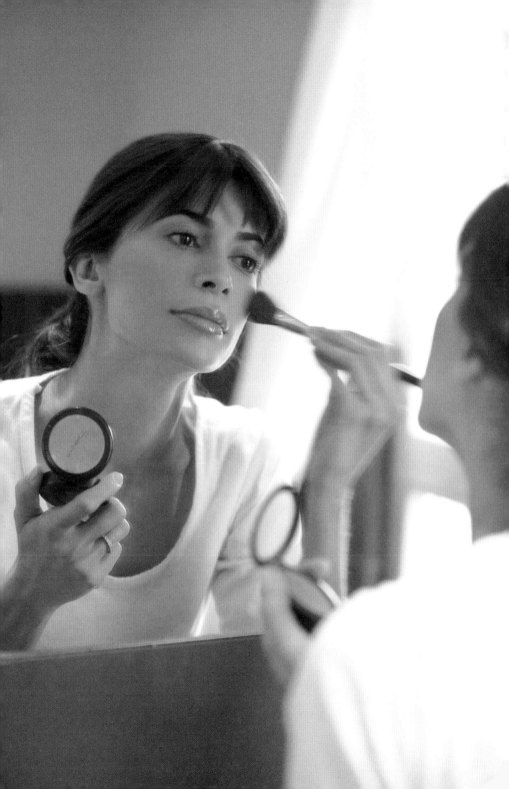

Eyeliner

Eyeliner is used to define your eyes and is applied very close to the top and/or bottom lashes. For a daytime look, a top line is sufficient, using a brown or light liner to naturally accentuate the eye. At night, you can use a bolder colour – black, blues and greens can be fun. You can apply it to the top and bottom and for a really defined look, try using a liquid liner.

Eyeshadow

Select a colour that will suit your skin tone

Warm skin tones – black, cream, bronze, light browns, soft greens and corals

Cool skin tones – whites, silver, pale blue, purple, dark green and greys

Eyeshadows can be tricky to apply, so if you're not entirely confident applying them, take a 'less is more approach' and add little bits at a time. There are a variety of application brushes you can use depending on the overall result you want to achieve.

The purpose of eyeshadow is to create contours and shadows around the eye to accentuate the eye shape. Fairly neutral colours will enhance your natural eye colour and can be blended with eyeliners to create a smoky look. During the day, use fairly neutral, light colours sparingly and blend well. For the evening, colours can be bolder and more dramatic. You can even add a bit of shimmer for a sexy glamorous look.

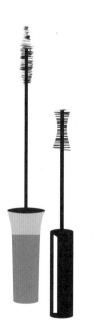

Mascara

Mascara completes the look of your eyes, and should be applied last. It thickens and defines your lashes, making your eyes appear larger. During the day, use a mascara from the brown family as this looks more natural. For evening wear, your mascara can be much stronger and darker – soft or jet black – to balance the darker, richer colours of your evening make-up.

Lip colour

Select a colour that will suit your skin tone

Fair skin tones – pinks, orange/red shades and light purples

Olive/yellow skin tones – browns, warm reds and very pale shades

Tanned skin tones – true pinks and peachy hues

Dark skin tones – rose, magenta and purple shades

There are three basic products designed for lips – lip liner, lipstick and lip gloss. A very natural lip liner is great for defining the boundary of the lip line, making lips appear fuller. It should always be blended in with either a lipstick or lip gloss so you can't see a defined line.

Lipstick will enhance your lips but choose a colour that works with your skin, as some colours are only suited to specific skin tones. During the day, stick to soft natural colours, but for the evening you can be more dramatic and use darker colours. Lip gloss can make your lips look fuller and more supple and will also give a more glamorous finish to your make-up.

Give it a rest!

Whenever possible, give your skin a breather and leave it free from any cosmetics or face products. Pores on your skin can often get clogged from frequent use of make-up, causing spots and skin irritations. I personally find that if you don't wear make-up for a few days, the next time you apply it, it looks even better than before!

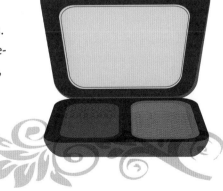

Make-up tips

In addition to the application tips on the previous page, here are some general make-up tips you might find useful.

- Remember the golden rule – make-up should enhance your looks, not overwhelm and consume them.
- Concealer, concealer, concealer – don't leave home without it!
- Avoid using foundation in the daytime – instead, apply a concealer to cover any dark circles or blemishes and use a soft powder to set it in.
- When applying make-up, always apply it gradually, because if you apply too much at the outset, you risk having to wipe it all off and start again. Too much make-up can also age you.
- For fast application and good coverage, try using a dual powder and foundation in one.
- Before applying your powder, try blotting your foundation with a tissue. This will remove any excess oils, and help to stop you from getting too 'shiny'.
- Focus a dominant colour on one area of your face and counter-balance it with a paler shade on other areas. For instance, if you choose a dark and smoky eye colour, use a light or more natural shade for your lips. Similarly, if you use a deep, dark lip colour, keep your eyes natural with the faintest hint of eyeliner or just a bit of mascara.
- Use an eyelash curler before applying mascara, or even if you're not wearing mascara. It will shape and curve your lashes, giving your eyes a 'wide open' appearance.
- To create fuller-looking lips, use a very natural pencil on the outer edge of your lip, be careful not to go too far outside, and blend inwards with a natural shade of lipstick or tinted gloss.
- Applying a soft rosy blush on the apple of your cheeks will give you a more youthful look.
- Shading under your cheekbones will enhance their definition.

How much you use depends on the shape of your face. Defining cheekbones too much can make some women look a bit chiselled and harsh.

- Highlighting the area just above your cheek bone and just under your eyes with a lighter shimmer powder opens up your eyes and lifts your cheekbones.
- Highlighting the top bridge of your nose with a lighter shimmer powder can refine and slim the nose.
- Blend your eyeliner with eyeshadow of a similar colour so the line isn't so sharp and severe.
- Use an old mascara wand as an eyelash comb – simply soak the wand in a liquid make-up remover and rinse and dry; it can be used again and again.
- Don't share make-up, especially applicators and brushes, as some skin conditions and eye diseases, such as conjunctivitis, are contagious.

Make-up must-haves

When it comes to your make-up bag, there are certain essentials every woman should have in it – the kind of things you'd want with you if you were stuck on a desert island! Here's my list ...

- Tweezers – to get rid of any last-minute stray hairs
- Make-up brushes – smaller travel-size ones are best to carry round
- Concealer – a must for blemishes and under tired eyes
- Powder/foundation – in a perfect match to your skin tone
- Eyeliner – to define your eyes
- Eyelash curler – to open your eyes up
- Blush – to give you a healthy glow
- Natural lip liner – to define your lips, or make them look fuller
- Lip balm/gloss – to keep lips soft, supple and sexy
- Moisturiser – in a sample size, in case of dryness or touch-ups
- Cotton buds – to touch up your face

Organise your make-up

How many of us have drawers filled with old dry make-up, with colours and shades we will never wear? How often do you keep make-up past its sell-by date without realising it? We are all guilty of hoarding make-up – me included! I've often been given the most extraordinary look for a photo shoot and thought how cool it would be to try and recreate it myself. I'd beg the make-up artists for samples or buy similar shades to add to my ever-growing collection. However, because it'd take forever to replicate, and was hardly appropriate for everyday life, I never got round to trying.

So, every now and then I purge myself of the 'vintage' collection of make-up I seem to amass – it's quite a cathartic experience. Give it a try yourself from time to time. Here are some tips that might help you.

● Keep it simple. This doesn't necessarily mean wear simple make-up, but rather get rid of make-up you don't or won't ever wear. Find the colours, shades and looks that suit you and stick to them. Throw the others away.

● Check the expiry dates on your cosmetics. Yes, make-up expires! You don't want infections from old make-up, so get rid of it. Aside from expiry dates, watch out for make-up which has dried out, smells rancid or with a changed consistency.

● Store your make-up in one place, ideally where you usually apply it. This way you can keep track of your collection.

● Try using a drawer divider to separate your lipsticks, blushes, eye shadows, etc. This will keep your collection tidy and allow you to see what you have.

● It's a good idea to buy duplicates of your everyday favourites and keep a spare in your handbag or at your office. This way you can touch up your make-up with identical products and also have a back-up if you lose something.

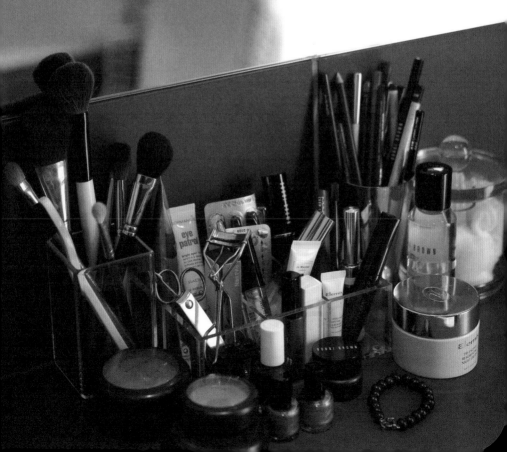

shelf-lives

→ Eyeshadow: up to 3 years
→ Mascara: no more than
  3 months
→ Concealer: up to 12 months
→ Foundation: 12–18 months
→ Eyeliner: up to 3 years
→ Lip liner: up to 3 years
→ Lipstick: up to 4 years
→ Blush: up to 3 years
→ Nail polish: 12 months
→ SPF lotions: 12 months

- You only really need a few make-up brushes to apply your make-up well. Invest in some good-quality brushes as they last longer and feel nicer on your face. My friend Jemma Kidd has an extensive range of great-quality brushes that fit perfectly into your handbag.
- Choose a tapered brush (rounded with a flat end) for lips and eye lining; a straight brush (bristles cut in an even line) for eyeshadow and eyebrows; and a chisel brush (bristles are slightly layered giving a rounded look) for blending.
- Keep brushes clean to prevent the build-up of make-up residue and bacteria. Wash in soap and water, then reshape them and stand them up in a cup to dry.

Hair removal tips

Hair removal – the bane of my existence, which I'm reminded of on an almost daily basis! I wish there was a precise, painless and hassle-free way of removing unwanted body hair but as far as I know it hasn't been discovered yet! Whether it's getting rid of hair from your legs, underarms, bikini area or eyebrows, it's a never-ending chore that most of us face on a regular basis. Maybe you want to try something for the first time or vary your methods of hair removal. If so, you might find this list useful.

And remember, don't be embarrassed when getting waxed in a salon – the person doing it has seen it all before!

→ If you don't tweeze or laser facial hair, you should bleach it; it opens up and brightens your face. (If you shave it, it will just grow back thicker and darker.)
→ Cleanse and exfoliate the areas from which you remove hair as much as possible to avoid getting in-grown hairs.
→ Avoid waxing and plucking during your menstrual period, as it will intensify any pain.
→ Waxing can be a better option than shaving, as the hair takes longer to grow back and can even start to thin.
→ To reduce pain of waxing, trim the hair first, take ibuprofen an hour beforehand and relax.
→ Don't shave with just soap and water. Use a good shaving gel, cream or foam and always use a sharp blade.

Method	Most effective areas	Pain factor	Cost
Waxing or sugaring	Legs, bikini, upper lip	Medium	Medium/High
Laser	Face and body	Medium/High	High
Electrolysis	Face and body	Medium/High	High
Shaving	Legs, bikini, underarms	Painless	Low
Epilators	Legs	Medium	Low
Depilatory cream	Body	Painless	Medium
Bleaching	Face and body	Painless	Medium
Tweezing/plucking	Face and other small areas on body	Low–Medium	Low

Dare to go bare?

The type of bikini wax you choose is down to personal taste and may change according to circumstance. If you're going on holiday and plan to wear a skimpy bikini, then you'd probably want to remove more hair than usual. But if you're preparing to reveal yourself for the first time to a new partner, then begin how you mean to go on! You're setting a precedent that you might not want to live up to on a regular basis, so you need to work out if all that pain (pure torture for most women) is really worth it. You can choose just how much or how little to remove, but here are a few of the standard wax jobs.

Basic bikini wax – Only removing hair from outside your knicker line.

The Brazilian – Contrary to popular belief, this popular wax is not totally bare, leaving either a small 'landing strip' or small rectangle or triangle of hair. Ideal for a very brief bikini, but also very painful!

The 'Playboy' – as seen on most *Playboy* models, like a 'Brazilian' but even briefer.

The 'Hollywood' or the 'Sphinx' – not for the faint-hearted, this is an everything-off wax, leaving you totally bare. The most painful!

Eyebrows

Plucking, or tweezing, your eyebrows can open and brighten up your eyes and face. But be careful not to over-pluck – too much plucking can result in a permanent mistake, with the hair follicles so damaged the brows can never grow back! It may be wise to get a professional to shape them first and then you can follow their outline by plucking as and when hairs grow back. If you prefer to do it all yourself, take your time, step back and appraise your brows each time you pluck a hair or two. Remember – taking too much off can leave you with a harsh and severe appearance.

And be sure to invest in a good pair of tweezers. Cheap ones never seem to work well and are very frustrating. I prefer pointed ones as they enable me to catch hold of even the finest and shortest hairs.

tips

→ If you have sensitive skin, pluck before bedtime so any redness will fade overnight. Otherwise, use good natural daylight to find all the hairs and see what you're doing.

→ Holding a pencil vertically along the side of your nose shows you where your eyebrow should start, and holding a pencil along the outside of the eye shows where the eyebrow should end.

→ Brush the eyebrow into place so the natural shape is neatly defined and you can see where to begin plucking.

→ Pluck below the brow, following your natural arch. Only pluck above the brow if there are any noticeable stragglers.

→ Definitely pluck any hints of a unibrow!

→ You will have less pain if you pluck close to the root and in the direction of the growth with one sharp and quick pull. Hold a hot towel over your brow for a few minutes to loosen the hair follicles.

→ Trimming also helps to define your eyebrows. Some hairs shouldn't be plucked because they would leave gaps, so if they are unruly use a pair of small nail scissors to trim them.

→ Fill in any gaps with a pencil or powder, using a shade close to your brow or even a shade lighter for a more natural look.

Hands and nails

It's important to take care of your hands because, other than your face, they're the most visible part of you. Your hands can give your age away, even if your face has had a nip or a tuck, so look after them before it's too late.

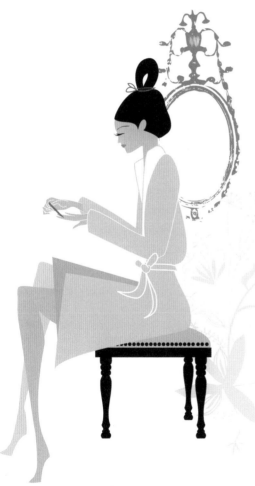

tips

→ Use a handcream as often as possible to keep your hands hydrated and moisturised. Keep some by the kitchen sink, some in your bathroom and place a tube in your handbag or car.

→ Try exfoliating your hands every now and again – you'll be amazed how smooth they feel afterwards. I exfoliate all the way up to and including my elbows. You don't need to spend a lot to get a good exfoliant – especially for the body. I use a wonderful one created by my friend Normandie, which leaves my skin feeling super-soft. Her skincare products are available in Tesco and are great value.

→ Cleaning products can do serious damage to your hands by stripping them dry. Use rubber gloves at every opportunity, even when washing the dishes.

→ Keep your nails clean and filed. It's quite off-putting when you shake hands with someone who has dirty nails!

The DIY manicure

What you need

varnish remover

soap

nail brush

nail clippers/
scissors and nail file

cuticle softener/
cream

bowl of warm water

cuticle stick

handcream

baby or olive oil

cotton wool

nail polish

base polish (if
using a dark colour
on top)

Keeping your hands looking clean, polished, and feminine doesn't require weekly trips to a professional. Give yourself a regular manicure following these guidelines.

1   Remove any old polish or dirt on your nails with varnish remover.

2   Give your hands a good scrub with soap and water or an exfoliator. Use a nailbrush to clean underneath and around the nail bed.

3   Clip and file your nails to the length and shape you desire. File only in one direction, not back and forth.

4   Apply a softener to your cuticles – use cuticle remover or a little cream, let it work in for a minute or two, then soak your fingers in warm water.

5   It's not good to cut cuticles so just push them back with the flat edge of a cuticle stick. If hangnails (little pieces of skin that can tear or snag) are present, carefully clip them. Use the pointed end of the cuticle stick to clean the grooves of any grime underneath the nails.

6   Apply a handcream and massage it into the skin and nails; you can even use some baby or olive oil to remoisturise the nails.

7   Clean the oil off the nails. Use a wooden cuticle stick with a bit of cotton wool twisted around the top, dip it into some nail polish remover and gently clean the surface of the nail.

8   Time to polish. Choose your colour carefully. Clear polish or light natural shades are ideal for everyday use and they also tend to last longer. You can be more adventurous with bold colours when going out.

9   Start with your little finger and work your way around. Apply the first stroke of varnish down the centre of your nail, then work outwards, taking care not to touch your skin at the sides. If you do, use the cuticle stick with varnish remover to remove smudges.

10 Apply two coats (not too thick), then apply a top coat (preferably a quick-drying one) to seal the colour and help it last. If you're using a dark-coloured varnish, you should put a base coat on first to avoid staining the nail underneath.

11 Don't touch anything for at least 20–30 minutes! (If you're having a professional manicure done, always pay for it before the manicurist starts, to avoid having to fish around in your bag for your wallet afterwards, thus ruining your nails!)

tips

→ To prevent a nail polish bottle sealing shut after use, wipe the rim of the bottle with varnish remover on a cotton bud.

→ Keep your nail polish in the fridge to make it last longer.

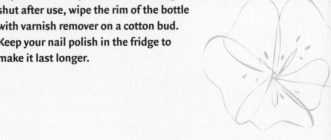

Heavenly soles and sexy feet

I get enormous satisfaction from wearing a pair of sexy strappy shoes or gorgeous summer flip-flops and admiring my newly pedicured feet. People either love or hate feet. I actually find well-maintained feet rather sexy.

The DIY pedicure

What you need

varnish remover

warm bath or tub of warm water

soap

aromatherapy oil

nail brush

nail clippers/ scissors and nail file

cuticle stick

pumice stone or foot file

foot scrub

flip-flops

base coat polish

polish

top coat sealer

In the summer, when your feet are most exposed, pedicures are essential. You can treat yourself by going to a salon, or you can do it yourself at home – I find it easiest and quickest to do in the bath.

1 Remove any old nail varnish and dirt with varnish remover.

2 Run a relaxing warm bath; add some aromatherapy oil to soak in and relax, if you have time. Keep your feet under water. If you don't have time for a bath, get a tub and soak your feet in warm, soapy water. Let them soak for at least five minutes. Use a nail brush to scrub away any dirt.

3 Apply a cuticle cream or oil to the cuticles and return to soak for at least another two minutes.

4 Trim your nails straight across and file to a square shape with a nail file.

5 Use the pointed end of a cuticle stick to clean any dirt or residue from under your nails. With the flat end of the stick, gently push the cuticles back and scrape away any softened dead skin. (I do this at least once a week, especially if I don't have a varnish on my nails.)

If you're doing your fingernails and toenails at the same time, do your pedicure first so you don't risk ruining your manicure.

6　Use a pumice stone or foot file to gently sand away the dry, dead skin on your feet. For extra softness exfoliate with a good foot scrub and rinse.

7　When you've come out of the bath or are finished with your foot soak, you should dry, then moisturise your feet with a foot cream (peppermint or tea tree are good for circulation) or use a rich body cream.

8　If you are going to varnish your nails it might be worth putting on a pair of flip-flops at this point, to avoid the risk of ruining your newly polished nails while walking around.

9　To varnish, first apply a base coat, then two layers of your chosen varnish and then seal this with a quick-drying top coat.

Haircare

Taking care of your hair is another essential part of your image. It's definitely something other people notice. Some days you may want to blow dry it, set it or create a look, yet other days you will choose your natural style. I have to admit that I often rush out of my house with my hair still wet and tied back. You aren't expected to create the perfect hairdo every day but even if you're going for the 'natural look', it's vital you look after your hair to keep it as healthy as possible and reduce the chance of breakage, split ends, hair loss, and dullness.

Shampooing and conditioning

To get 'clean and healthy' hair, you don't have to wash it every day. Leaving your hair a day or two between washes is generally best – indeed, my hair actually looks better the second day after washing. Use a good quality shampoo and conditioner as you may find the cheaper brands actually dry out your hair. If you have naturally dry hair, avoid using a shampoo and conditioner 'in one' as it won't provide enough moisture.

Many products are formulated with specific ingredients to suit specific hair types so check which ones are best for you. If you use a heat styling instrument such as a hairdryer, straightening iron or curling iron, make sure you use a leave-in conditioner to add moisture and offer a coat of protection from the heat.

Always rinse the shampoo and conditioner out thoroughly after each application and every couple of months give yourself an intense conditioning treatment, especially if you have coloured or damaged hair. I have an intense conditioning treatment at Daniel Hersheson's salon about four times a year, straight after having my hair coloured, and it leaves my hair incredibly soft and shiny and totally revived.

Cutting

Hair should be trimmed every six to eight weeks, although depending on your style and how fast your hair grows you may need a trim every four weeks. If you're considering a change of image and feel like a new hairstyle, consult with a hairstylist first. Different styles will suit different face shapes and ages. You should also consider whether the style will complement your overall look, from head to toe, including wardrobe, makeup and general style. Think carefully before making drastic changes as it will take a long while to grow back out!

Colouring

Unless you use a pretty solid one-tone colour, I'd leave colouring to the professionals, especially if you're thinking of highlights. It's difficult to produce natural looking highlights and I've even had colourists get it wrong! If you insist on doing it yourself, buy a really good hair-colouring kit and follow the instructions precisely to avoid any mistakes. Again, think very carefully if you are considering a complete colour change. Make sure it will complement your skin tone and natural features.

If you highlight your hair, it's best to go only up to four shades lighter, as this prevents the colour looking harsh and unnatural. It also reduces the appearance of different-coloured roots when your hair starts to grow. This also applies to lowlights, where you may be bringing your hair colour down slightly.

Protect your hair

Sun can damage your hair, making it dry, brittle and bleached, so if it's going to be exposed to the sun for a long period, cover it with a hat, wrap or scarf. There are plenty of products on the market to minimise the damage, such as intensive conditioners.

Chlorine can damage and dry out hair too. If you swim regularly, wear a protective cap if possible. If not, shampoo and condition it immediately after swimming. Remember – don't swim within a week of colouring or highlighting your hair, as the chemicals might react and change the shade of your hair. Some highlights have been known to turn green!

Vitamins and minerals

There are several vitamins and minerals that help keep hair in good condition, including vitamin A and B. Eat plenty of yoghurt, eggs, green vegetables and bran products and perhaps try a supplement. I occasionally take a vitamin supplement called Perfectil, which is formulated for hair, skin and nails, especially if I feel my hair is looking particularly dry and dull. Minerals such as zinc, iron and copper are also good for your hair and are found in most forms of protein and green leafy vegetables.

Detangling

It's best to start with a wide-toothed comb when trying to detangle your hair, especially if it's long. Gently start at the ends and work your way up towards your scalp. Detangling wet hair is very difficult, so brush your hair before you wash it to avoid having to comb out knots afterwards.

Blow drying

When using a blow dryer to style your hair, use a brush to create tension and hold the hair taut, thus stretching it into a new shape. Heat can damage your hair so don't aim the blow dryer on one spot for more than a few seconds.

Straightening

You should always begin straightening your hair with a hairdryer first, then polish it off with a good pair of straightening irons to give it a sleek look. Never use straightening irons on wet hair – it will burn it. Finish the ends off with a light gloss or sheen to control any flyaways – add a little to your fingertips and comb it through.

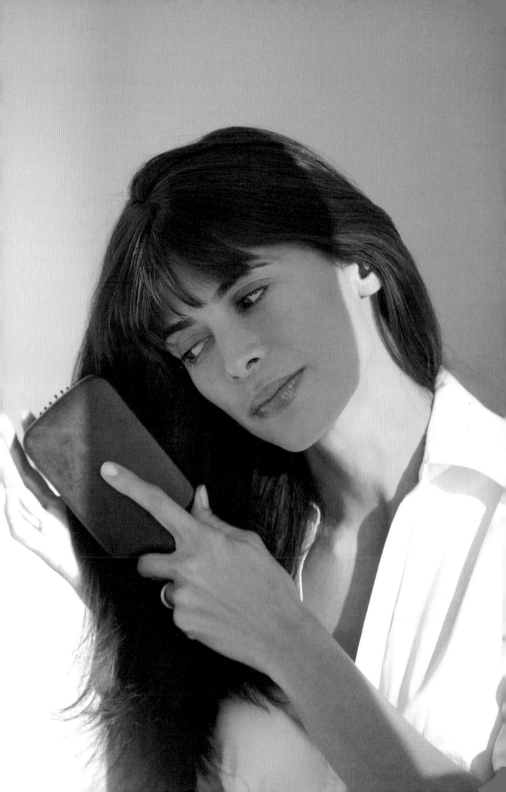

Cushion-style brush – A flat-backed brush with a bed of bristles on what looks and feels like a cushion. Best for medium-length hair that is naturally smooth and straight.

Paddle brush – A wide, flat brush – great for brushing and blow drying long hair and for creating straight, smooth styles. Not good for adding volume, or for using on layers.

Metal-based or thermal brushes – These are best for conducting heat and creating shape, making styling easier.

Round brush – Best for smoothing hair and flipping ends out or up and creating volume.

Sculpting brush – Great for backcombing to add volume to short, textured styles that need some movement. Best for short cuts, round layers and textured outlines. Think of choppy ends and razored perimeters.

Combination nylon/bristle brushes – Good for curly or coarse hair – the brush eases through hair, causing less stress on the strands.

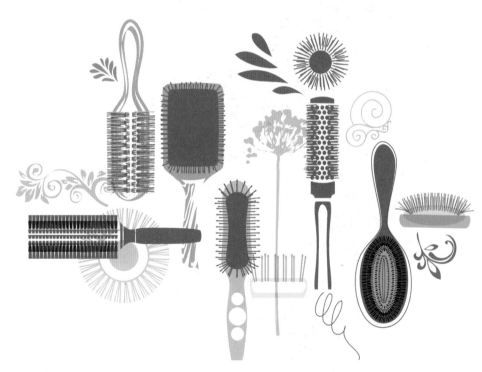

Hairstyles

Having healthy hair gives a big boost to your overall appearance, but equally, so can your hairstyle – a different cut can completely change how you look. So how do you decide what will look great on you? If you're considering a new haircut, first have a think about the shape of your face and your hair texture.

The shape of your face

A hairdresser once showed me this quick and easy way to figure out my face shape.

1 Stand in front of the mirror and tie your hair back, keeping all short wisps of hair back with a headband.
2 Using an old lipstick, draw around the outline of your face in the mirror. Step back and look at what shape you've drawn.

Once you've decided what face shape you have, use the guide below to work out what styles are likely to suit you the most.

Round

A round face is circular shaped, with the length approximately equal to the width. Try a below-the-chin or shoulder-length hairstyle worn straight and close to the face. Centre partings are best. Avoid curls and hair on your forehead.

Heart-shaped face

A heart-shaped face is wide at the forehead and cheekbones, but narrow at the jaw line. To reduce the width of your forehead and make your jaw look wider, try soft and curly chin-length hairstyles. A chin-length or short bob is great for creating a balanced look. Avoid short top-heavy cuts, full hairstyles or slicked-back looks as these will emphasise your upper face.

Oblong face

An oblong face is longer than it is wide. Try any short to medium style because too much length will make an oblong face look even longer.

Oval face

With an oval-shaped face, the length is equal to roughly one-and-a-half times the width, and the forehead and jaw are of similar width. Most any hairstyle will look good on you! Wavy, straight, curly, long, short or medium hair lengths. You should experiment and see which one you like the best.

Long face

This face shape is longer than it is wide, with a long straight cheek line. Chin-length bobs and cuts are good for long faces. A fringe or wispy hair on the forehead would look good, but make sure the cut is not too top-heavy. Avoid extremely long or short cuts as these will make your face look longer. If you want to have very long hair, try adding a few long layers.

Square face

Square-shaped faces are angular and have a jawline, cheekbone and forehead that are almost equal in width. Medium to short length hairstyles will be best for you, especially with a wave or cut that comes around the face. Soften the edges of your face with layers and try a side parting. Avoid tying your hair back tightly or having square, geometric cuts, long bobs with heavy fringes, or any style that includes a middle parting.

Triangular face

Triangular faces tend to have wide chins and narrow foreheads. Try shorter hairstyles that balance your prominent jaw line, with lots of layers angled towards your chin to achieve fullness and balance in the upper part of your face. Try parting your hair off-centre and avoid long full hairstyles and styles that add width, such as haircuts that kick out at the bottom.

Your hair texture

Fine or thin hair – can look very good in a blunt cut. Try keeping it short or shortish, and perhaps use a chin-length cut.

Coarse or medium hair – can handle a lot of styles, although it might be best to avoid a very short cut, as it can look bushy and stick out.

Thick or heavy hair – would be better kept at a medium or long length as it might not hang very well if cut short.

Golden glow

We all feel good with a golden glow on our faces and our bodies but the damaging effects of the sun's ultraviolet rays make it very dangerous to lie in the sun to achieve this look. In fact, the skin tans to protect itself from further damage so it's not actually a sign of good health at all. Exposure to the sun can cause irreversible damage to your skin, making it appear saggy, leathery and deeply wrinkled. It can also lead to different types of skin cancer, which together form the most common type of cancer in the UK, with the malignant melanoma leading to 1,700 deaths each year. Whatever your skin tone, everyone is at risk. So perhaps now is the time to consider alternative tanning methods!

The sun is a good source of vitamin D, but you only require fifteen minutes of sun a day to encourage your body to produce enough vitamin D to keep your bones and immune system strong. Just by walking around you absorb all you need. If you need to be outside during hot weather, use a high factor suncream and cover up any areas that are continually exposed. No matter what protection you use, avoid lying in the sun for extensive periods of time.

And don't be fooled into thinking sunbeds are a safe alternative. They still emit ultraviolet A (UVA) rays, which penetrate into the deep layers of your skin. They cause damage even before your outer skin layer appears red, meaning you're not even aware of the harm.

There are many self-tanning products available these days to give you colour without any risk of UV exposure. But remember, when faking it, less is definitely more – aim for a golden hue rather than an all-over orange glow!

If a healthy glow is all you want, invest in a bronzer. Take time to choose the best colour for you; ones with a hint of shimmer are especially great if you're going out at night. Apply your bronzer with a specialist bronzing brush to achieve an even application. The most common places to highlight with a bronzer are the face, neck, shoulders and cleavage.

For an all-over tan, you can choose to 'do it yourself' or go to a salon. Until recently, a tan from a bottle or a salon could leave you looking like a carrot, but products have progressed immensely and are now easy to use and give you a natural-looking, wonderful tan. Self-tanning products range from sprays to gels, lotions, wipes, and even a pill. If you're nervous about applying it yourself, opt for a spray treatment at a salon. It's quick (about 30 seconds!) and gives you an instant even tan with no mess.

tips

→ Exfoliate your skin before applying a self-tanning product.

→ Don't shave your legs just before application.

→ Try to apply it before you go to bed to give it time to set overnight – but make sure you wait long enough so your sheets don't turn orange!

→ Rub the product into the skin thoroughly – every nook, cranny and crevice!

→ Rub around your wrists and the back of your hands to blend the tan in with your arms, and into your ankles and the top of your feet to blend in with your legs.

→ Don't forget! Wash your hands with soap and water after applying the product to avoid ending up with bizarrely tanned hands.

→ If you make a mistake, try using hydrogen peroxide, which you can get in most pharmacies. It will lighten dark spots and remove stains from your palms. Make sure you rinse it off thoroughly afterwards.

I find the best way to do your own self tanning treatment is to have a bath a bit before bed, exfoliate your body, apply the tanning product, and put on dark pyjamas so as not to risk staining them. Then I can shower again in the morning to remove that funny smell that some tanning products have. Saying that, I've recently found a product which gives a great natural tan and it doesn't have any strange smell. It's called Xen-Tan and it gives you a deep tan in three hours, which is very helpful when you have a last-minute wardrobe change and want to expose a bit of leg!

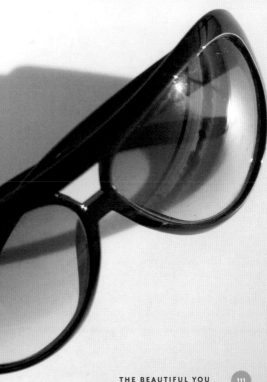

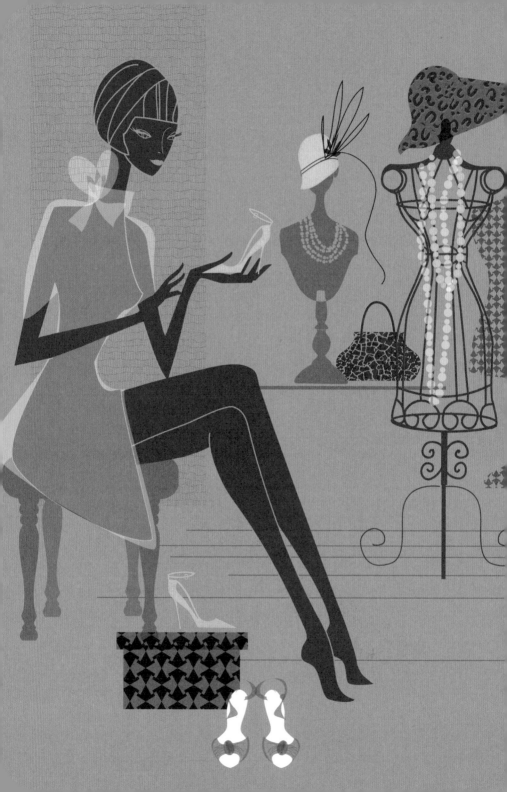

the 5 stylish you

'Fashion fades, but style is eternal.'
Yves Saint Laurent

This spot-on statement straight from the mouth of one of fashion's great icons is something we should all bear in mind when choosing our wardrobes. While fashion comes in waves and trends, style is more personal, and less superficial and transient. The essence of style comes from within.

Having style is all about having a look that is unique to you. It's about understanding your own characteristics – colouring, height, body shape, personality – and knowing how to make the most of these elements so you look good and feel great about yourself. It also encompasses the impression you make on others, which comes from your sense of self – for the truly stylish, this will shine through whatever fashion they choose. Remember – you have the power to give every outfit your own unique touch.

Style

Being stylish is not as simple as spending vast amounts of money on designer brands and keeping up with trends. In fact, inexpensive clothes can be worn with style as long as you know how to make the most of your natural features. Equally, expensive clothes will look completely unstylish if they are not right for you. To create your own style with almost anything to hand, you just need a good eye for detail and a bit of thought. I remember finding a long, flowing, rose-coloured dress at a charity shop and instantly falling in love with it. I pinned a similar, but slightly deeper-coloured chiffon rose at the bosom and wore it to a glamorous red-carpet event. To my delight, the outfit received countless compliments and when a TV presenter asked me who the designer was, I took great satisfaction in replying: 'Not sure – cost me £5 from a Cancer Research shop!'

'Fashion can be bought. Style one must possess.'
Edna W. Chase

One of the golden rules about style is that it should appear effortless, without seeming false or strained. Remember – not every fashion trend will suit you, so don't force yourself into an impulse purchase just because fashion magazines tell you to. It can be handy and fun to be aware of current trends, but the most important thing is to feel comfortable with what you wear and only adopt a particular look if it's right for you.

tips

→ Think impact

→ Maximise your assets

→ Wear clothes that are the correct size and fit well

→ Know the clothes that flatter you but don't be afraid to experiment

→ Carefully consider what kind of occasion you are dressing for

→ When in doubt, keep it simple

→ Don't disregard an outfit just because someone else doesn't like it – if you genuinely feel good in it, chances are you look good too

So how do you know for sure what's right for you? This is a tricky one, but as long as you're aware of your own body shape and best features – you're on the right track! You can also ask a trusted friend to go through your current wardrobe with you, and take them along on shopping adventures for new additions – make sure it's someone who has their own sense of style that you respect. You also need to feel sure they'll give constructive and honest opinions about what you wear. This should help you to be open to new ideas and looks that might work for you, but ultimately – always trust your own instincts. It may take some trial and error and lots of looking in the mirror, but it'll be well worth the effort.

Just because an item of clothing comes with a designer label, doesn't necessarily mean that it's stylish or even of particularly high quality.

Dressing with style

Dress for the occasion

Concentrate on the impact you are trying to make and what message you want your appearance to send out. If you're going to a particular event, always check if there's a dress code, and choose your outfit accordingly. If not – you need to assess the type of occasion yourself and decide what you think will be appropriate. On a day-to-day basis, be realistic – while you don't want to look scruffy, a pair of sexy high heels is never the right look for a trip to the supermarket or walking the dog!

Be aware of your body shape

Make sure you know which parts of your body to draw attention to and which parts you want to hide. Learn to appreciate clothes that flatter you and accept that others do not. Always wear clothes that hang well whether they're tailored or a relaxed fit.

Wear your size

Be honest with yourself and wear clothes that are your real size – it's actually much more flattering. Don't hide behind too-loose clothing, but by the same token, don't try and squeeze into something two sizes too small either. Either way you could make yourself look bigger than you actually are – by hiding your shape or by spilling out of something that just doesn't fit. It's important to know your measurements too – so take a moment to measure all the key parts of your body (hips, waist, bust, leg length) and put them into your phone or diary so you have them when you're out shopping. If you know a good tailor, then consider getting certain pieces of clothing adjusted, for a perfect fit.

Taking your measurements

Stand in front of a mirror, either naked or with very light clothing on, and use a dressmaker's measuring tape to measure (without pulling too tight) around the following points:

Hips – measure the widest part of your hips and bum

Waist – measure at the smallest circumference of the tummy

Bust – measure just under your armpits and over fullest part of your bust

Leg – measure the inner length of your leg, remembering to add extra height for any heels

Consider your age

You may still fit into that gorgeous little mini you wore when you were eighteen, but it doesn't mean you should wear it now. Dress your age! The good news is that 40 is the new 30, 30 is the new twenty, and so on – so dressing your age can still be fun and sexy.

Know what colours suit you

Colours can be divided into four groups – named for the seasons. You can find out what group of colours is most flattering to you by working out what 'season' you are, going on your eyes, skin and hair tones. I fall between two seasons – autumn and winter – meaning most colours from both suit me – but I should also avoid wearing certain colours from both categories. The good news is we generally innately choose colours which suit us, as these tend to be our favourite colours. If you're not sure, use the chart opposite to see which category you might fall into, and play around with different colours in front of a mirror to see what works with your skin. And don't panic if you see that a colour you love isn't meant to flatter you. No colour has to be entirely banned from your wardrobe – perhaps try keeping it away from your face, or combine it with one of the colours which most suits you. Go on, have a go – it's great fun!

	Skin tone	Hair	Eyes	Flattering colours	Colours to avoid
Autumn	golden, olive, beige, golden brown and ivory	brunettes, auburn, redheads, blonde, copper, black, grey	brown, dark and deep, hazel, green, blue/green, turquoise	earth tones: dark brown, mustard, beige, rust, gold, olive, forest green, teal, turquoise, mauve, orange	yellow, light grey, pink, black, blue, red
Winter	olive, yellow, dark, black, pale white	brown, dark brown, ash brown, black, silver grey, white	brown, dark and deep green, deep blue, hazel	primary colours: navy, black, white, red, grey, taupe, fuchsia, mauve, turquoise, purple, lemon, burgundy	rust, brown, beige, gold, orange, peach
Spring	creamy white, ivory, beige, golden, pink or peach	golden blonde, strawberry red, blonde, golden brown	blue or green, golden brown	red, yellow, orange, beige, peach, light blue, violet, bright green, pink, ivory, white, camel, tan, golden and light browns	black, dark brown, blue-red, blue
Summer	pale or pink beige, ruddy, pink, rosy-brown	natural blondes, brunettes, ash blonde, silver, brown (mousey), pearl white, platinum, dark brown	blue, light eyes, grey-green, grey, soft brown, hazel, aqua	pastels, navy, white, blue-green, grey-blue, pink, lavender, plum, aqua, yellow, rose, greys	orange, gold, black, yellow-green

Top flattering styles

- Svelte style – wear one colour from top to bottom – black is the most slimming of all
- Stripy style – vertical stripes are more flattering than horizontal ones running around your body

- Symmetrical style – if you have a small upper body and larger lower body, wear light colours on top and dark colours on the bottom, and if you have a smaller lower body than upper, try the opposite
- Self-assured style – avoid feeling self-conscious by covering up problem body parts such as tummies and upper arms

Know your body shape

We all know we should dress to flatter our figures. The key is to work out what styles ultimately show off our best bits, and just as important – disguise our least favourite parts. Nobody's perfect, and all the women I know have something about their body that they'd like to change. After two babies, I'd certainly like to change the way my stomach and breasts look!

But by accepting our 'problem bits' and loving our best features, we're on the road to finding our own style – we just need to accept that some trends will never suit us, no matter how up-to-the-minute they seem!

It's amazing the countless shapes of women's bodies. This means that many women don't actually fit the mould of 'standard' body shapes such as pear, apple, hourglass, full-figured and slender. This means it can be more helpful to understand the style solutions for specific problem areas instead.

Short legs

With short legs, your best trick is to create the illusion of a longer leg.

→ **long wide-legged trousers** – long enough to hide your shoes; high heels or platforms will elongate your legs
→ **wear long skirts** – again, when worn with heels, this gives your lower body length
→ **wear Empire-line dresses** – the style comes in at the bust, rather than the waist, disguising where your legs actually begin

→ tight, cropped or high-waisted trousers; these shorten your legs
→ tight-fitted dresses that show where your legs begin, emphasising their shortness

No waist

It doesn't matter whether you're stocky or have a flat, taut tummy – you still might yearn for more of a waist. Here are some ways to create more of a waist, or alternatively, to draw attention away from that area.

→ wrap sweaters, blouses and dresses – they give the illusion of pulling in a waist
→ small prints on your blouses and dresses that pull focus away from your waist
→ corset-like tops pulled in at the waist
→ belts that pull in the waistline
→ tailored jackets with tight waists

→ baggy shapeless tops or blouses
→ shift dresses, the shape is too square, giving you the appearance of no waist
→ high-waisted trousers or hipsters

Chubby tummy

Chubby tummies are a tricky one for women, especially after childbirth. While it's not necessarily easy, this one is at least fixable if you step up your exercise and watch your diet. In the meantime, here are ways to disguise your belly!

→ a girdle to pull everything in, giving you a smooth stomach with support and control
→ Empire-line styles that skim over the tummy area
→ Ruched tops that hide some of the folds of the tummy

→ tight-fitting trousers, hipsters or skirts that give you muffin-top; your stomach will just hang over the waistline.
→ tight belts – your tummy will squeeze out both over and under it
→ short crop tops or blouses which expose any flesh
→ stretchy or clingy dresses and tops – as these will certainly reveal a flabby tummy

Big bosoms

If you have big breasts, the biggest worry is looking too top heavy or tarty. If you choose clothes in the right style and fit, though, these can be your biggest assets (excuse the pun!).

- → good supportive bras in a variety of styles so they can work with your entire wardrobe
- → wide necklines, which are very flattering on the neck
- → tops and blouses which fit snugly around the waist area, with a looser fit around the breast
- → corset types of tops
- → wrap tops, cardigans and dresses
- → V-neck tops

- → halter-neck tops or dresses – you can't wear a supportive bra
- → high-necked tops and T-shirts, which make your breasts look even bigger
- → sleeveless tops and blouses
- → thick knitted sweaters – they'll make you look bigger than you are

Small breasts

The great thing about small breasts is that you can easily make them look better when you want to. The other advantage is that certain styles will suit you better if you have small rather than big breasts.

- → the right size bras
- → added pads or gel inserts for an immediate size boost – make sure your bra will accommodate them
- → high or scoop necks
- → one-shouldered vests, blouses, tops and dresses
- → sleeveless tops
- → thick knitted jumpers, polo necks and cardigans
- → Empire-line styles that are ruched around the breast area, giving the appearance of fuller breasts

- → cuts which are too low – as there's not much to display!
- → dresses which are skin tight up top
- → corsets – you've got nothing to fill them with!

Thick ankles and calves

If you have thick ankles or calves, you've probably already realised there's nothing you can do to change them. Don't worry – there are plenty of tricks to keep them well hidden!

- long skirts as they'll completely hide the shape of your lower leg – or if you want to wear a shorter skirt, choose a knee-length A-line cut, which gives the illusion of a thinner leg
- long trousers – wide-legged or flared are your best options as these don't cling to your leg

- trousers that are cropped above the ankle – this will emphasise a thick ankle
- shoes which have a strap around the ankle, as these again highlight the width of your ankle
- ankle boots which emphasise your large calves

Big thighs

If you carry extra weight on your thighs, or if you have particularly large thigh muscles, there are lots of things you can try out so your top and bottom halves look balanced.

- flared or wide-legged trousers to create a straight line down the length of your leg and balance your lower legs with their top halves
- A-line cuts in dresses and skirts
- one-shouldered tops and wider necklines balance out the thighs and hips
- a dress over trousers – great for hiding those saddlebags

- straight leg or drainpipe trousers which show that the upper and lower halves of your legs are unbalanced
- bias-cut dresses or skirts – the worst cut you can wear if you are also pear-shaped, as it really accentuates your bum and thighs
- large or bold prints
- jackets or coats which sit on the widest part of your hip
- high tight-waisted trousers

Big bum

Women with big bums can use many of the same tricks used to disguise big thighs. Remember that a shapely, curvaceous bottom can be very sexy (think Beyoncé!).

- tailored and fitted skirts and dresses – if you want to outline your bum
- loose-fitting trousers – if you want to hide it
- jackets that cover the bum

- A-line anything – this style flares out in the back, making you look bigger than you are
- short jackets which end at or above your bottom – your bum will look big and wide in comparison

Classic style – wardrobe essentials

There are some items every girl should have in her wardrobe, regardless of current trends. This is what I call a capsule wardrobe – a set of reliable basic fashion items that you can mix and match for every occasion. This collection of timeless clothing forms the backbone of your wardrobe and can take you from season to season.

It's definitely worth investing in some classic garments, so spend as much as you can afford on key items that you will use over and over again. The use you get from them will far outweigh the cost and they can easily be mixed with less expensive 'this season' items to create a trendy look.

Your capsule wardrobe overall will save you time and money – it simplifies your life and helps ensure that when you walk out your door you are looking your best!

When choosing a party dress, a simple classic timeless style that flatters your figure can make as much of a statement as something over the top. Fussy only ever looks fussy! You can always accessorise with a gorgeous 'wow' piece of jewellery to give it more life.

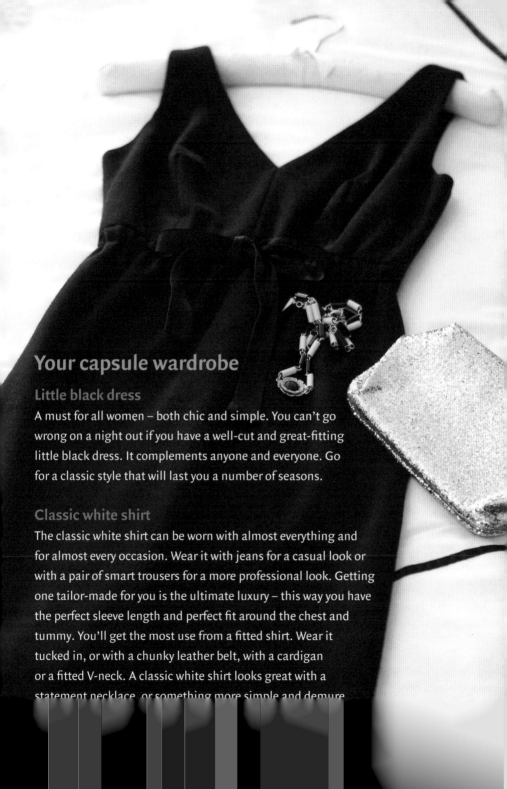

Your capsule wardrobe

Little black dress

A must for all women – both chic and simple. You can't go wrong on a night out if you have a well-cut and great-fitting little black dress. It complements anyone and everyone. Go for a classic style that will last you a number of seasons.

Classic white shirt

The classic white shirt can be worn with almost everything and for almost every occasion. Wear it with jeans for a casual look or with a pair of smart trousers for a more professional look. Getting one tailor-made for you is the ultimate luxury – this way you have the perfect sleeve length and perfect fit around the chest and tummy. You'll get the most use from a fitted shirt. Wear it tucked in, or with a chunky leather belt, with a cardigan or a fitted V-neck. A classic white shirt looks great with a statement necklace, or something more simple and demure.

Great-fitting jeans

Jeans are probably the most versatile garment in your wardrobe – you can wear them everywhere – both for day and night and for casual and dressy. If you find the perfect cut of jean for your shape, it's worth buying two or three pairs if you can afford to. Lighter denim looks relaxed for more casual daywear, while darker denim is great for taking you from day to night. Choosing a denim which has some stretch means your jeans will keep their shape better. Hems are also an important consideration – for jeans to be properly stylish, the hems should be long enough to almost cover the heel of your shoe. Similarly, if you're wearing flats for a more casual look, make sure you're not treading on your hem (don't roll your jeans up!).

Fitted jacket

A great fitted jacket has multiple uses. It can be worn with a smart shirt and trousers, or just with a pair of jeans and T-shirt. When choosing a jacket, the key is to find one that fits the widest part of your body really well. You can have the rest of it tailored and taken in if necessary.

tips

→ choose a high-quality fabric
→ choose a cut which suits your shape
→ if having one made – get both skirt and trousers to match the jacket

Tailored suit

A woman in a well-cut suit looks incredibly stylish. Suits nowadays not only look very sophisticated and professional, they can also look super sexy. These days, suits can be worn almost anywhere – for meetings, interviews, dinners, cocktail parties and even big social events. Having one tailor-made will ensure the best cut and fit, but if you want to spend less, high street stores produce amazing suits as well – find the cut which suits your shape, buy the best quality you can afford, then have a few alterations if needed.

Black trousers

You can't go wrong with a pair of well-cut black trousers. Choose the style that suits you best, and these will be incredibly slimming and flattering. Black trousers can be worn both for day or night, casually, for work, or for a dressy occasion. A wider-legged trouser looks very chic when partnered up with a sexy blouse, camisole or fitted jacket. Longer hems worn with heels will elongate the legs and look incredibly sleek and stylish.

Timeless skirt

Choose a simple style in black or grey, so it works with almost everything. An A-line cut suits most figures, but a great-fitting pencil skirt can look sophisticated and sexy. Accesorise a skirt with coloured or textured tights, take a skirt from day to night by changing sandals or flat shoes for a pair of sexy pumps or strappy heels, or stay warm in winter with some stylish knee-high boots.

Cashmere jumper

There's nothing better than the feel of a soft and cosy cashmere jumper or cardigan. Aside from their comfort and warmth, they also look very chic and are great for day or evening. These are a worthwhile investment – a good-quality jumper lasts a long time if properly cared for, and the classic styles never go out of fashion. To dress it up, wear it with tailored trousers or a stylish skirt and add a silk scarf or jewellery, or for a more low-key look, combine it with jeans.

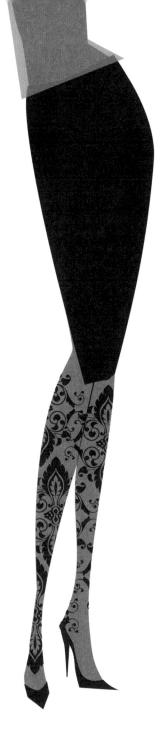

Cashmere is traditionally known as super-expensive, but you can get great bargains now through places like Tesco, M&S and GAP.

Classic coat

A great coat is an essential garment that completes most of your winter wardrobe looks. Stick to a classic colour for more versatility – black, grey or navy blue.

tips

→ look for a perfect fit – you shouldn't be drowning in excess folds, nor should it be too tight
→ check you can cross your arms in front of you and reach up comfortably
→ consider what tops fit comfortably underneath – do you have room for that extra layer?
→ choose a great quality fabric – one that will withstand heavy wear and tear and won't wrinkle easily

Statement pieces

Despite the practicality of a capsule wardrobe, every now and again all women need to make a statement. For this reason, no wardrobe is complete without a few signature pieces. These can be pulled out of the closet when you want to make a grand entrance and stun a crowd.

Statement pieces don't tend to be great value for money as they lose their impact if you wear them too many times. So because they aren't a fashion 'need', I always try to buy my special items during the sales and hang on to them until that special occasion comes along – saves me time and money in the long run!

- Choose bold, large patterns or geometric prints on beautifully cut dresses and blouses. Try starting with subtle colours and work your way up to bold and beautiful as your confidence grows.
- Choose rich fabrics like velvets, tweeds, chiffons or silks to up the ante of a look. Metallic fabrics also have a lot of wow power.
- Choosing a piece in a strong colour, like a red, fuschia or jade green, can look stunning.
- Fine detail such as beading, sequins or layered fabric, ruffles or ruching can give a piece of clothing that something extra. Don't go overboard though – make sure any detailing or bold colour is balanced by simplicity in some other areas – like the cut.

Shoes

I absolutely LOVE shoes and boots and can't get enough of them. One of the reasons so many of us have such an obsession with shoes is because there's an endless variety to choose from depending on the season and event – and you can always find something to express your personality. Slipping on a pair of strappy heels or sexy pumps can change your look completely, from day to evening, while metallic leathers add a bit of sparkle and go with nearly everything.

When it comes to buying shoes, don't skimp – spend as much as you can afford. A lot of people say you can judge a person by their shoes, and your shoes do affect the overall impression you make. Better quality shoes are generally more comfortable, look more stylish and last longer too.

Here are a few of the classic staples that will see you through any occasion. With all of these in hand, you can start investing in more unusual, fabulous and eye-catching shoes that you could just die for!

Everyday shoes

When choosing shoes for day-to-day wear – consider the comfort, fit and style. Neutral colours (brown and tan) and black are most versatile and will go with everything. Leather ballet-style flats are great everyday shoes – they look great with jeans, skirts and dresses, worn casually or when dressing up.

Pumps

A high-heeled close-toed shoe is a definite classic staple for your wardrobe. This simple timeless shoe has a wide variety of styles and shapes, but choose a slim heel with a rounded point for the most versatility. Invest in a great quality black leather pair, and if your budget can afford it, look out for a neutral-coloured pair as well.

When opting for a pair of killer show-stopping heels, try gel inserts. They'll save the balls of your feet a lot of pain, and you won't need to walk home barefoot at the end of the night!

High heels

A dressy black high-heeled shoe for the evening is every woman's wardrobe prerogative. Strappy is always sexy, as long as it's not too chunky or heavy! Aside from a gorgeous black pair, it's also a good idea to invest in a gold and a silver pair of strappy evening shoes. Between the three of these, you'll have something for every outfit.

Trainers

Trainers have come a long way, and these days are incredibly designed with fashion sensibility in mind. I live in them during the day, not only because they offer great comfort (something you need when chasing around two kids!), but they can look really stylish with what I am wearing.

Boots

A winter essential; invest in a great everyday flat boot in black leather or brown. For evening, a knee-high boot with a heel looks great with most everything.

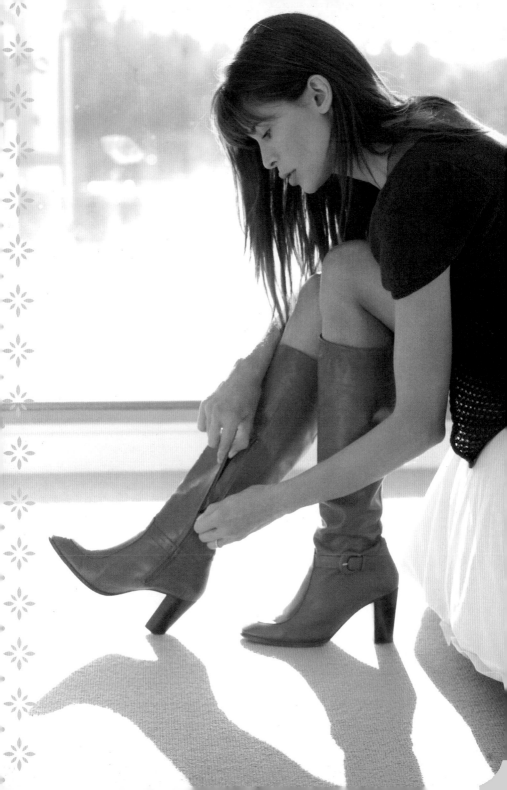

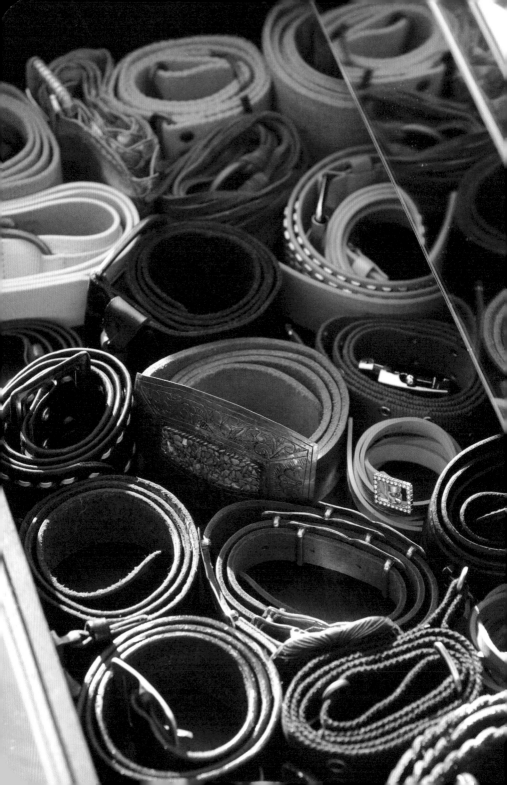

Accessories

There are endless accessories you can use to add to the look of an outfit, including jewellery, belts, hair clips, wraps, sunglasses and handbags. If you're adventurous and confident, accessorising is one of the most fun parts of defining your style – it brings your look to life! Accessories can define your individuality; and have the power to change a relatively plain or simple outfit into something unique and special, and can even enable you to wear the same base layer for more than one occasion.

Don't get too carried away though, and if in doubt, keep it simple. I had a girlfriend in LA who thought just because all of her accessories were individually stylish and wonderful, she could wear them all at once and look fabulous – let's just say, she looked like a walking Christmas tree!

In general you should only use two or three colours at a time and try not to be over-bold or too loud. The best way to get new ideas is to people-watch and decide what looks good on others, then give it a try yourself. It's easy to get away with inexpensive jewellery and other accessories – look out for great sales in high street stores like Accessorise, where you can pick up some amazing bargains.

tips

→ Consider the combination of everything you are wearing from head to toe – this includes your sunglasses, jewellery, belt, handbag and shoes

→ Everything you wear should be complementary and not clash

→ Balance the size and proportions of your accessories with the type or style of clothing you are wearing – don't wear platform sandals with your business suit, or drag along a big bulky handbag with an elegant evening dress

→ One standout accessory makes more impact than a number of less memorable ones

→ You can get away with inexpensive jewellery, but bags and shoes should always be of the highest quality you can afford

Jewellery

Jewellery is an easy way to add glamour to your outfit. Try a pair of large hoop or ethnic-inspired earrings with your hair tied back to add a bit of chic to your look. Layers of funky beaded necklaces look great when added to a simple white shirt or plain dress – very boho chic. Lots of mixed bangles are also eye-catching. Diamonds certainly have wow appeal, but don't over-bling it – you risk looking tacky and downright vulgar. I feel that if you've got some major bling, then it deserves to be worn on its own as a special piece – so it stands out and gets the attention it deserves.

As a general rule, I usually choose to wear either earrings or a necklace, and not both at the same time. Be aware too of how your jewellery ties in with your clothes. Certain cuts of blouses, tops and dresses – ones which expose lots of neck or shoulder – allow you to make a statement with a chunky beaded necklace, or a big piece of bling. On the other hand, if you have a busy neckline or one with lots of fabric covering the neck, opt for statement earrings instead.

Evening bags

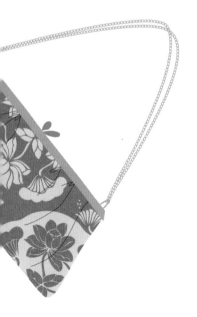

When trying to dress up a plain or classic outfit, you can be a bit more adventurous and opt for a sparkly evening bag, but if you're already wearing a statement outfit, it's better to go for something simple. A clutch bag is the perfect accessory to complete your evening look – incredibly elegant and chic. It should be big enough to carry your evening essentials, yet small enough to hold in your hand; it has clean lines and understated details. There are an enormous variety of clutches out there – leather, metallic, beaded, woven – and luckily, unlike big everyday bags, you don't need to spend a lot to find a great-looking one.

Scarves

A small or delicate scarf is a great accessory for both day and night. A patterned silk scarf worn tied around the neck with a classic white shirt looks hugely sophisticated, or you can team a thinly woven metallic one with a black blouse for evening. Woollen winter scarves are mostly worn with coats, but can also complement a big woolly jumper.

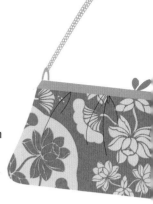

Wraps

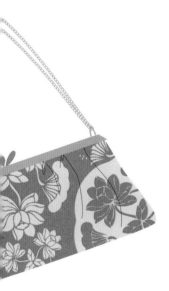

A wrap or shawl not only keeps you warm, it can also finish off a look. They look great worn casually, or if for more dressy occasions, drape around your bare shoulders over a strapless dress. I pack at least two whenever I travel, not only for warmth and comfort during the plane journey – they're perfect for tropical holidays when it may get cool in the evening. Having at least one black and one neutral (like a beige or cream) wrap will prove invaluable additions to your wardrobe – they go over everything. After that, the range of colours, textures and patterns is endless and a vividly coloured wrap can look stunning over a simple outfit.

In the office

Unless fashion is your business, you should play it fairly safe when accessorising yourself for work, especially in an office environment – bling is definitely not the thing here! You can still wear a wonderful piece of jewellery or handbag, but keep it understated and simple to keep yourself looking as professional as possible.

Underwear

We often forget that your underwear is also a chance to express your personality – a little bit like shoes – but in secret! The variety available is amazing – there are so many colours and designs, and bras and knickers can be sexy, fun, playful or sophisticated, as well as strictly practical.

Because you wear your bras and knickers underneath your clothes, it's also easy to forget that they make a huge difference to your outward appearance – so a good fit is essential.

Unsightly lines, bumps and bulges are too often the result of bad underwear and can be easily avoided. It's also important for both support and comfort to have a well-fitting bra, so make sure all your underwear is the right size and shape and get rid of the rest!

Bras

Your breasts can change size significantly through pregnancy, menopause, weight gain, weight loss, when taking a contraceptive pill, and sometimes even for no reason at all! With this in mind, it's a good idea to have your measurements taken every two to three years. Most large department stores and lingerie shops offer a free fitting service but if you prefer to measure yourself, try this guide.

- Measure in inches around your body under your chest – where the bottom of your bra would sit comfortably
- Add 4 if it's an even number and 5 if it's an odd number to get your band or back size
- Measure in inches your bust size at the fullest part of your breasts, pulling the tape as tight as is comfortable
- To find out your cup size, deduct the band size from the bust size
- If it's the same, you're an A cup, if there's 1 inch difference, a B cup, 2 inches a C cup, and so on (to be even more specific, use double letters for half-inch differences)

tips

- try seamless bras and knickers for their smooth appearance – great under fitted clothes
- use strapless bras with strapless dresses and tops
- use double-sided tapes with low-cut dresses and tops – where no bra is humanly possible!
- if you have prominent nipples, consider wearing a slightly padded or moulded bra – especially if your top is fitted or sheer
- wear nude underwear if your clothes are sheer – invest in a selection of nude bras and knickers – as they'll all come in useful at some point
- always wear G-strings with tight-fitting trousers and skirts
- remember to wear low-cut thongs or knickers under hipsters – a whale-tail poking out the top looks tacky beyond belief
- wear fuller knickers or French-cut knickers when you wear loose-fitting dresses or trousers
- always check for VPL (visible panty line) in the mirror before you go out!

It's smart to buy more than one type of bra, depending on what you're wearing. For example, if you're in a strapless dress and are not comfortable going without a bra, you'll need a strapless one. Or if your clothes are sheer, you should wear nude-coloured undergarments so they're not noticeable. And if you're exercising, you need a bra that provides extra support.

With these tips in mind, it's wise to invest in a collection of staples – nude, black, padded, seamless, push-up, strapless – that take you from day-to-day wear to every different clothing occasion. But once you've dealt with the practicalities of your underwear, it's time to head out and have fun. A vast array of underwear in all styles, colours and materials is waiting for you, so go on, indulge yourself!

A camisole looks great worn alone or under a blouse, dress or jacket. It's also great as lingerie!

Take stock and get organised

OK – now you've assessed your personal style, you've probably got some ideas on how you'd like to change or add to your image. So how do you go about evaluating the clothes you have already to see what you need to buy?

1 **Take stock and clear out**
2 **Organise your wardrobe**
3 **Put on your shopping shoes!**

A good place to start is by taking stock of what you have in your wardrobe. We've all stood in front of the mirror endlessly trying on a range of garments to see what looks best for a date, a job interview or that special occasion, but this is actually a very good way of assessing what you have!

Your aim is to have several basic clothing pieces you can mix and match to make a variety of outfits. Think about what type of clothing you need, including a range of casual, smart and best outfits, based on your job and your lifestyle. Be honest with yourself and get rid of anything that doesn't suit you or no longer fits. Be brutal – and think about quality over quantity. You can take your unwanted clothes to charity shops, or arrange an afternoon tea for your friends, where you can all swap the clothes you no longer wear.

Almost every woman battles for space in her wardrobe, so doing a regular overhaul is a liberating and cathartic experience – think of it like a spring clean. I do a full clear-out once a year, but continually weed during each season to keep my closet from heaving. You can turn the messiest area into a wonderfully functional closet. A well-balanced wardrobe that uses space efficiently makes it much easier to get dressed in the morning – and more importantly, it gives you the perfect excuse to go shopping for the things that you're missing!

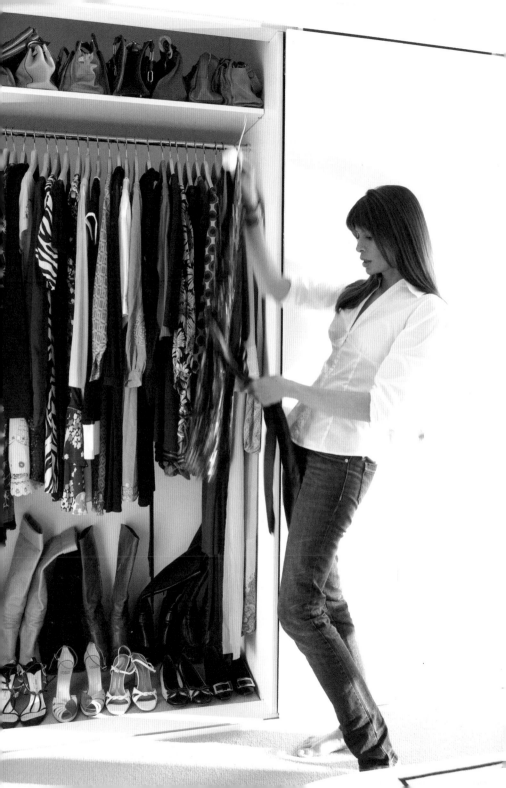

- Only keep clothes which fit well, look good and give you confidence – they should complement your best physical features and be in colours which suit your hair, eyes and skin tone.
- Get rid of clothes you haven't worn or thought about in over a year – unless they are wonderful designer pieces that will stand the test of time. These more special pieces can be stored away until they come back into fashion – automatic vintage clothing!

Organise your wardrobe

Once you've got rid of everything you don't need, it's time to get organised! Having your clothes in order allows you to select your outfits properly every single day, and also makes sure you make full use of all the items in your wardrobe.

- Put together your capsule collection of fashion basics – your 'Definitely Can't Live Withouts'! These stay in your closet year round and should take prime positions for easy accessibility and use.
- Rehang these according to type of clothing and length – dresses, shirts, trousers, skirts etc.
- Categorise other areas in your closet – for instance, if you're sporty, keep all your sports clothes together, or if you travel a lot, have a section for the items that travel well. Select an area for your work clothes and for your play clothes.
- Move special event outfits and showstoppers to the back of your wardrobe – although they're probably your favourite garments to have on display, you don't need to access them on a regular basis.
- Trim down your closet for the current season. Move seasonal items to the front of your closet and store the rest until the weather changes. Make sure you always have on hand the items which cross over between seasons.

If it helps, create a wardrobe inventory to organise and itemise your clothes, including shoes, handbags, belts and scarves, as well as your jewellery. This is a good way of keeping track of what you actually have, especially if you pack away your seasonal clothes. Go to my website for a template – www.lifestyle-essentials.com

● If storing any clothing, make sure you do so carefully – use protective clothing bags and then hang in a storage closet or pack into plastic boxes. If storing woollen garments, include a moth repellent – I like using cedar chips rather than ordinary moth balls because they smell lovely.

Storing accessories

Shoes – Storing shoes can be a real problem – but I still don't think you can ever have too many! Lots of different storage systems are available – including racks, hanging compartments and clear plastic shoe boxes. Or keep the shoe boxes they come in and stick a picture of the shoes on the box.

Belts and scarves – Try rolling in shallow drawers, or buying a special belt hanger. Small storage boxes can also work well for these.

Handbags – Try a long shelf at the top of your closet, where you can line up your bags according to colour and size. For smaller evening bags, try a specific drawer or small storage boxes.

Care for your clothes

Your clothes are an investment and if you want them to last a long time and keep their shape, you will need to care for them properly. I know I've ruined too many of my favourite clothes by washing them at the wrong temperature!

- Always follow the washing instructions on the care label
- Turn delicate clothing inside out when ironing and double check the temperature
- Use plastic or wooden hangers rather than wire so your clothes keep their shape
- Make sure that skirt/trouser hangers have a protective clamp that won't mark your clothes

Caring for leather

Leather is a natural fabric and will last for years if cared for properly. If you've got any fine leather clothing or expensive delicate handbags, or if the leather has unusual or extensive stains, then I'd highly recommend letting experts clean them.

If doing it yourself at home, then leather is best maintained by cleaning gently by hand at least twice a year. Follow the steps below for general leather goods – including shoes, bags and belts.

1 Use a mild soap or saddle soap to create suds in a bowl
2 Apply the suds (not soapy water) to the leather surface with a soft cloth or sponge
3 Keep the sponge barely damp and not wet, as some leather will stain or change colour if exposed to too much water
4 Clean quickly before any fluid can soak in or dry on the leather
5 After cleaning, buff dry with a second soft cloth
6 Don't leave to dry near heat, as the leather can become brittle and possibly shrink
7 After drying is complete, rub in a leather conditioner to protect from spills and stains and keep the leather soft and supple

When storing leather items, remember that any extremes in environment may damage the surface or cause the colour to fade. Keep leather goods in a cool area out of direct sunlight where air circulates so it can breathe. If the item has a suede finish, keep it covered so it can't collect dust.

Time to shop

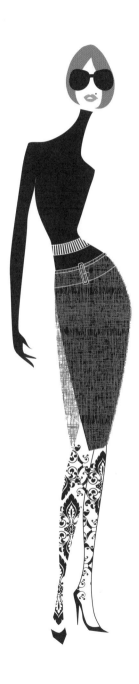

Now that you've identified what you have, it's time to identify what you need in order to complete the style you desire. There's no need to break the bank if you look for things that will go with more than one item you already have, automatically giving you several new options. Or could you buy a few accessories to brighten up existing items? It's always better to fill the gaps in your current wardrobe rather than trying to buy an entire new one!

Once you're confident about any new clothes you need and the style that you want, it's time to hit the shops. Most importantly, always bear in mind your lifestyle and buy clothes that realistically work for you. While sales are a great way to pick up a bargain, it's important that you don't buy something just because it's 'on sale'. If it's not something you'd normally pay full price for, then make sure you really like it and will actually wear it – and that you're not just buying it because it's cheap!

If you're shopping for an extra special outfit for an important occasion, or find something that's more expensive than usual, take your digital camera – this lets you take a picture and review it again later, or show it to a friend for their opinion.

Most importantly, keep your capsule wardrobe in mind, and if you want to stay ultra-focused while shopping, write down the clothes you're looking for before you start out. If your list is long, prioritise each item in case you run out of time and can't get everything on the same day.

Shop til you bop

Shopping on your own can be great, because it lets you focus entirely on what you want – no waiting for other people to queue for changing rooms! But shopping with someone else can be great fun and hugely helpful too – just make sure it's someone whose sense of style you admire and who you trust to be honest with you rather than polite.

Whether you have specific items in mind, or are simply in need of some retail therapy, here are a few of my top shopping tips to make it through the day.

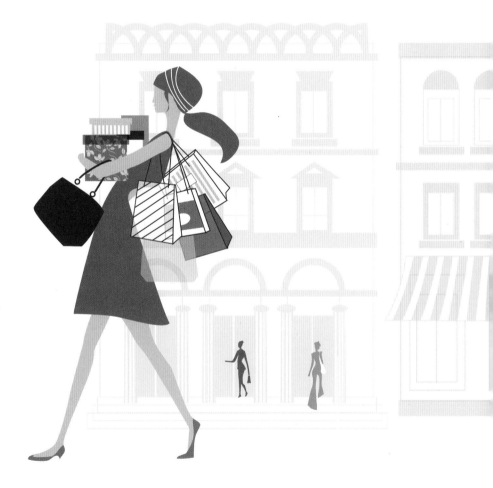

- Don't shop on an empty stomach – without energy, enthusiasm and a clear head you might make a decision you later regret.
- Wear comfy shoes. There's nothing worse than tired, sore and aching feet while tramping from shop to shop. Avoid laces, or tight boots, as they take too long to put on and off.
- Wear easy on–off clothes – you don't want to spend all day sweating as you struggle in and out of a tight outfit.
- Wear a well-fitting bra and knickers as they affect the overall image of the outfits you're trying on.
- A G-string is generally better as it reduces the chance of a VPL (visible panty line) and is hidden under any item of clothing.
- Don't be intimidated by pushy sales staff – you have every right to take your time and browse in any shop. If they hover and push items on you, politely tell them you wish to look for yourself.
- If you're on a tight budget or just can't find what you are looking for, try a secondhand or charity shop. You never know what bargain you might find!
- Try before you buy – I always do. Sizes for women's clothes vary greatly between stores and brands. Even when the queue stretches for miles – remember how much more of a hassle it will be to return it another day.
- Beware the skinny mirror. Enough said!
- Check the return policies when paying and keep the receipts and tags of everything you buy until you've worn them. Sometimes you get home and decide something doesn't look as good in your own mirror, or match an outfit as you planned.
- If you find something you absolutely love that's perfect for you, consider getting it in other colours, or even buying two of the same.

Online shopping – for my favourite shopping links, head to www.lifestyle-essentials.com

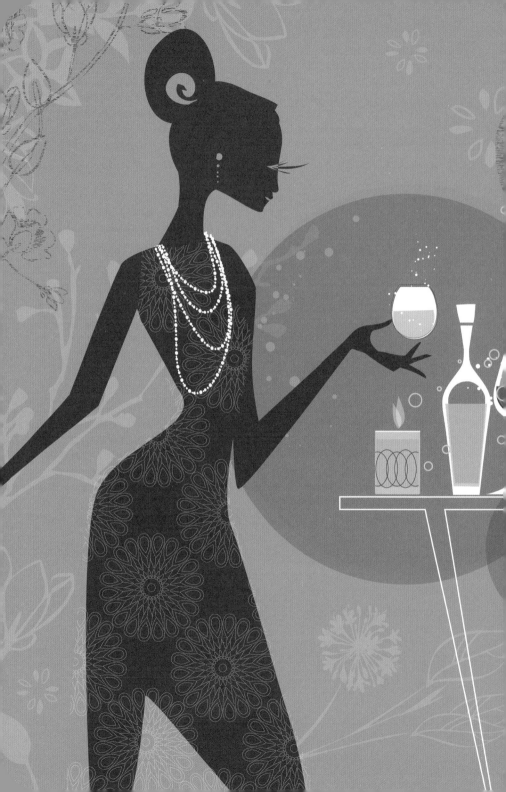

the charming you

6

First impressions are incredibly important – and although the first impression you make on others is definitely affected by how you look and how you dress, these are not the only factors. You also need to consider how you behave towards people. This takes a key part in shaping the way you are seen and influences others' conclusions about your personality. Some of us are born with natural charisma, but for those of us that weren't, it doesn't mean you can't attain it!

By being charming you'll be certain to make a good impression wherever you go – by delighting, attracting and fascinating others. Charm is the ability to set others at ease, while also making them feel they are interesting and important to you.

In the old days, women would be sent to finishing school to be taught the intricacies of being a domestic goddess. Society's moved on a long way since then, but this doesn't mean that we should fail to be charming and gracious while also following empowered lives. Charming people have the warmth and confidence to draw others towards them, and this is a great skill to apply in all spheres of life – both personally and professionally.

In this chapter we'll look at many different forms of being charming – common courtesy, how to communicate well socially and at work, and how to charm the pants off a first date! We also uncover the secrets of being the hostess with the mostest, and equally important – the perfect guest.

The courteous you

One of the most important forms of charm involves courtesy and consideration for others. For me, manners are synonymous with respect – for oneself and for others. Having good manners is principally about being a decent person – about being kind, considerate, polite and behaving appropriately in different environments.

We'll look more closely later at some manners specific to particular social occasions, but to start with here's a quick list of essential basic manners – do a check to see which you already always practise, and if there's any you might need to work on a little.

- Be respectful – Treat others the way you'd like to be treated yourself.
- Be punctual – It's inconsiderate to keep people waiting, especially if they're on their own.
- Be polite – Remember to say please and thank you, no matter who you're talking to. Always knock before entering someone's room or office.
- Be discreet – Cover your mouth when coughing, sneezing or yawning. Don't talk too loudly in public, especially on your mobile.
- Be thoughtful – Offer your seat to an elderly or pregnant person, or someone with a disability. Don't smoke around others without first asking if it will bother them.
- Be gracious – Learn to apologise. Admitting you're in the wrong and saying sorry can be hard to do but it stops resentment and bitterness from escalating.
- Be cheerful – Smile! It costs nothing and could cheer up others as well as yourself. It takes four times as much energy to frown as it does to smile.

'All people smile in the same language.' *Anonymous*

The art of communication

Interacting easily with others is definitely a skill we should all try to perfect. Almost every situation you find yourself in requires some form of social interaction, so how you react to others and how well you communicate are definitely essential in all aspects of life. Every time you open your mouth you reveal something about yourself to the person you are speaking to, in exactly the same way as you reveal your personality through your body language, as discussed in **The Essential You**.

The art of communication may come naturally to some, but not to all of us. Talking to others, particularly to those we don't know very well, can be nerve-wracking – none of us want to appear boring or uninteresting and all of us want to make a good impression, though without appearing over-confident or arrogant. By learning how to engage others in two-way conversation we can gain enough confidence to be able to handle any situation, professional, social or otherwise, with aplomb.

'Good communication is as stimulating as black coffee and just as hard to sleep after.'
Anne Morrow Lindbergh

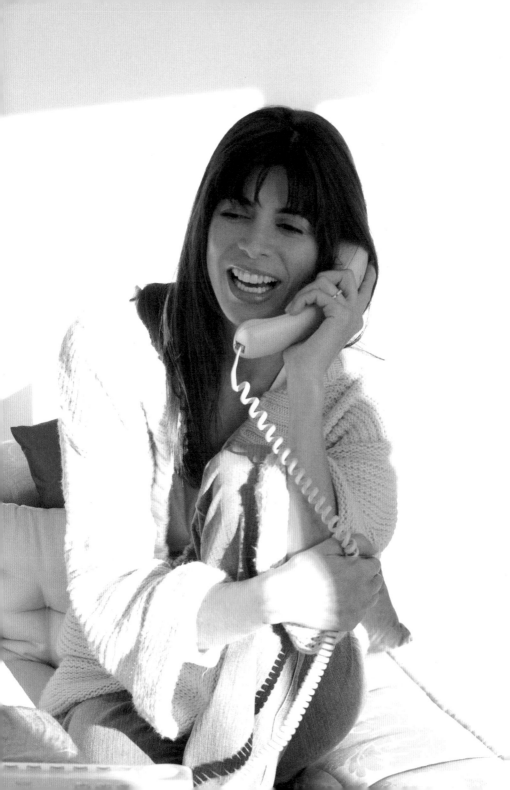

My useful tips

- Remember names – repeat the person's name when you're introduced and, if it's unusual or difficult to pronounce, ask them how to spell it to make sure you've got it right. To lock it into your memory, use their name as often as possible in conversation.
- Remember one thing about each person, or who introduced you – this helps you remember the person for the future and gives you an immediate opener for your next conversation. If I'm given contact details, I always jot down this extra information.
- Give the person speaking to you your undivided attention and show a genuine interest in what they are saying.
- Maintain eye contact and don't fidget or look elsewhere while someone else is talking.
- Always speak clearly and sincerely.
- Ask questions when you don't understand something, rather than just nodding in agreement. It draws you into the conversation and shows that you've been listening and are interested.
- Be aware of people who are being left out of a conversation, or contributing less, and draw them in by asking their opinion or advice.
- Make yourself heard but don't shout, interrupt or talk over others.
- Don't always talk 'shop' or stick only with subjects you are familiar with, as this limits the number of people who will find you interesting. Make an effort to learn about current affairs and a range of topics so you can contribute easily to different conversations.
- Be complimentary where deserved but don't be too eager to praise – it can appear patronising and not genuine.
- Avoid being confrontational or aggressive – try to defuse heated conversation rather than encourage an argument – even if you think you are right!
- Remember – most people find it easiest to talk about themselves, so if conversation is becoming strained, ask a question about the other person.

Office etiquette

Within the workplace, as everywhere else, good manners and basic consideration will always serve you well. There are also a few other key points to address to be sure you're the epitome of charm and courtesy in the office.

Appearance

Depending on your profession, you should be well presented – always dress suitably and be clean and neat when in a work environment.

Phone etiquette

Good phone manners are extremely important – they can make or break your professional image.

Answering the phone – Always let the person know who they've reached – politely and clearly state the company name, or your own name on your direct line.

Taking messages – If taking a call for another person, always offer to take a message and don't forget to pass it on!

Mobile phones – Change your ring tone to vibrate whenever possible in any professional environment (and the same goes for public places). If you must take a call, excuse yourself and go to another room to take the call.

Email etiquette

As formal letters are gradually dying out, so the importance of email etiquette is ever growing. Email is a wonderful invention, but only if it's used properly and with care – many people get themselves into all kinds of trouble that could easily be avoided.

- Emails often get lost in cyberspace, so never assume an email has been received and read by the intended recipient, especially if it concerns anything significant. Request confirmation, and if none is received, phone to check it got through.
- Avoid giving bad news or firing someone by email.
- Unless it's necessary for recipients to see who has been copied in, use the BCC facility to protect others' addresses, especially when drafting a mass email.
- Don't send joke/bulk mail to or from your work account – save that for your personal email accounts. Bear in mind that some people get hundreds of work-related emails a day, so don't clog up their inboxes.
- If you're in disagreement with someone and have drafted a harsh email, leave it for a while if possible. Reread it once you've cooled down and before you press the send button. Once it's sent, it can't be retrieved.
- Do spell checks!

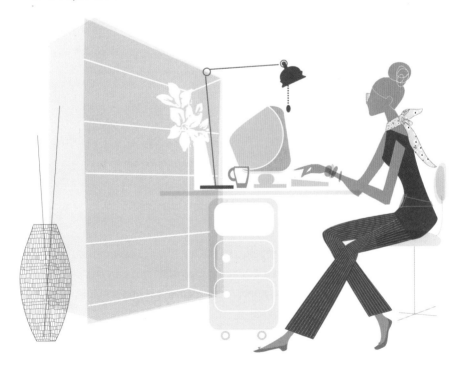

Dating

There are countless relationship gurus out there who believe that dating is a world of very complicated dos and don'ts, but I don't buy it. I believe dating should always be fun – and at the very least, they are opportunities for new experiences and to meet new people, even if it turns out a particular date wasn't right for you.

Before I met my future husband, I was never particularly good at knowing when someone was into me, nor at consciously flirting with men. But I have always really enjoyed meeting new people – I tended to live in the moment and simply enjoy chatting to them rather than trying to read something more into it. If you really fancy someone, I think this is the best way in any case – engaging in conversation and getting to know them a little better.

Initiating conversation can be difficult and can certainly make you nervous, but if you can overcome that and feel confident in yourself, you may just meet the person of your dreams or a friend for life.

Developing your natural charm is a way of meeting people you might be interested in, and then in making sure the first dates get off to the best start possible. And realistically, many first dates could possibly remain just that. But if you are truly charming, when you're not interested in taking things further, you'll be able to let a date down graciously and on good terms – with the same courtesy that you'd hope a man would show you.

How to meet someone

Stay open to potential venues for meeting people – it doesn't have to be a party, bar or club; it could be the park, the gym or even the supermarket.

● Create opportunities where you can casually talk to someone without it feeling like you're chatting them up. Don't come on too strong – it can come across as as pushy or intimidating and be offputting.

- Avoid using cheesy chat-up lines – yuck!
- Remember that less is more – keep them intrigued. Once you've engaged your potential date in conversation and got their telephone number, don't overstay your welcome.

First date charm

Once you've secured that first date, now's where the panic and anxiety can really take hold. Funnily enough, although I was useless at recognising the potential for a date, once they were actually organised, I always loved first dates – I found the possibilities they held so exciting. While there are no surefire rules, there are a few things you can do, both before and during the date, to carry off your dates with charm, style and flair.

Before the date

One of the most crucial elements of a good first date is getting the venue right. If you're arranging to meet someone, but you're not entirely sure whether it's an 'official' date (maybe only one or the other of you has romantic intentions) – it's best to start with meeting for coffee or lunch, as they have a clear timeframe. This way there's no pressure on either side to stick around if it's not going fantastically.

Personally, if I was going on a first date with someone I really liked, I'd always choose to go to dinner, and suggest a restaurant with good food, of course, but also where I knew the lighting was good (very vain, I know, but it is a first date!). It's good to be able to enjoy a nice glass of wine too – not something I would at lunch. Having a drink or two can help ease anxiety and lets you relax into your date. Just remember – stick to a couple of drinks – getting even remotely bevvied isn't very attractive and can lead to undesirable outcomes!

Wherever you go – make sure it's somewhere you feel comfortable and relaxed, which is not too noisy – so you can enjoy getting to know each other without having to shout!

Here are a few other tips on what to do before the first date

Be safe – If you don't know much about the person you're going out with, choose a meeting place with lots of people around. Leave the details of where you'll be with a friend, housemate or family member, along with the time you're expected home. Don't go home with your date, or invite them home with you, until you've really got to know them.

Dress appropriately – Obviously, you want to look your alluring best. But best doesn't mean overtly sexy, excessive bling jewellery or tons of make-up. Classy and stylish, with simple elegance is what you want to go with. And make sure you choose the right clothes for your activity – for instance, avoid heels on a picnic!

Be well-groomed – Clean everything – need I say more?

During the date

By being both interested and interesting, you can charm any date and save yourself from any potential awkward silences. It's better to establish common ground first before moving to topics such as politics and religion where you might disagree, so give yourself lots of topics to talk about by beefing up on current affairs, or talk about a great film or book you've seen or read lately. Remember to share the conversation as well – ask your date questions and listen with genuine interest. Explore the things you do have in common, as these may pave the way to meet up again. And don't reveal intimate secrets or talk about ex-boyfriends – it's only the first date!

Be on time – No one likes to be kept waiting, and doing it on a first date starts things out on the wrong foot – it sends out the message that you consider your time more important than his.

Enjoy yourself – Be positive and happy – it should be fun!

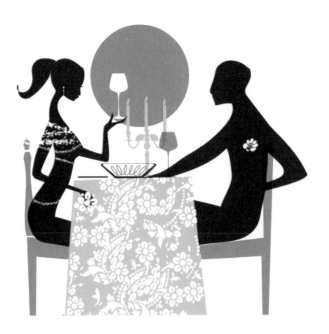

Body talk – Be aware of your body language. Almost every facet of our personality is evident from our appearance, posture and the way we move. To show your interest, lean in a little, use hand gestures to show animation and keep eye contact (but don't stare too intently!). Smile often – if he knows you're enjoying his company, he'll immediately find you more attractive.

Be open and non-judgemental – Don't jump to conclusions and judge your date on one thing alone – give him a second chance and work out what your overall impression is. Remember, your date may be just as nervous as you!

Be complimentary and thoughtful – Everyone likes to be told they look good – and it will instil confidence in your date. While you're out, be attentive – your date should feel that they are the only person in the room. Flirting with the cute waiter is a definite no-no.

Put sex on hold – Getting to know each other is always best before jumping into any form of intimacy – sexual or otherwise; the anticipation can only add to the excitement when you feel you are ready, too!

Being a gracious guest

I have to say that I find that the most gracious guests are those who've had plenty of practice at being hosts themselves – and who fully appreciate the effort it takes to host events, dinners or weekends. When I was single, I was forever the guest and it was great fun. Now that I'm married and have a house in the country, we tend to host more, and although I have an equally great time, it can also be exhausting and time-consuming.

When you're enjoying someone else's hospitality, it's important to show your gratitude by being charming and well-mannered and acknowledging your hosts' efforts – whether the event is a dinner party, a picnic or a stay in their home. Over the countless social occasions I've attended and hosted, I've seen both the best and worst of manners in guests, and here's what I've learnt …

General tips

- If you receive an invitation that asks you to RSVP, do so as promptly as possible – ideally within two days.
- Note down any dress code and if in doubt ask – we've all seen the fancy dress scene in *Bridget Jones's Diary*!
- Don't arrive early, and let your host know if you're delayed for any reason. If you can't make it at all, never simply fail to show up.
- If in doubt about anything, always ask – don't assume.
- Muck in – be positive and helpful, and get involved with the activities your host has planned.
- Offer to lend a hand with things like serving dinner and clearing or tidying up.
- Show your gratitude by complimenting your host's efforts.
- Don't overstay your welcome and know when to call it a day!
- Depending on the occasion, bring a gift to show your thanks, or send a thank-you card shortly afterwards.

At the table

One of my biggest pet peeves is poor table manners. Good table manners are a way of making sure your dining companions don't feel uncomfortable, and showing respect. It's easy to slip up and forget the odd one occasionally, so here's a quick refresher list of dining dos and don'ts!

DO

→ arrive at least fifteen minutes before dinner is being served, unless told otherwise

→ put your napkin on your lap when you sit to eat

→ sit up straight, don't slouch and keep your elbows off the table

→ only start eating when everyone has been served

→ use cutlery from the outside and work inwards

→ spoon soup away from you and tilt the bowl away too

→ break off a small piece of bread or roll at a time and butter each piece rather than the whole slice

→ eat at a leisurely pace

→ try to make sure you talk to both people sitting next to you

→ excuse yourself when leaving the table

→ compliment the cook – even if the food wasn't great, they've gone to the effort of cooking you a meal!

→ always say please and thank you, especially if people are serving you

→ if you don't like something you've just taken a bite of, discreetly spit it into your napkin and dispose of it when you can

→ when you've finished eating, place your knife and fork side by side in the middle of your plate, with the fork tines up, knife to the right and blade turned in towards the fork.

DON'T

→ make a fuss about where you're sitting or rearrange place cards

→ put personal belongings on the table, such as phones, bags, sunglasses, etc

→ smoke while people are still eating – and always check if anyone minds before lighting up

→ rock back in your chair

→ apply make-up or comb your hair at the table

→ overload your plate with food – you can always go back for seconds

→ talk with food in your mouth or chew with your mouth open

→ reach across the table – ask the closest person to the item to pass it to you

→ use your fingers to push food onto your spoon or fork

→ interrupt others while they're talking

→ stuff your mouth with food – keep your bites small

→ wave utensils in the air, especially knives

→ pick your teeth at the table, even with a toothpick – excuse yourself and go to the bathroom

→ push your plate away when you've finished eating

Being a good houseguest

If you're actually staying at someone else's house, then all of the tips above come into practice. But along with these, there are a few specific things to be aware of.

- Respect the routines of your host.
- If there are house pets, find out how they're allowed to behave – if they're allowed on furniture, to go outside, to have treats, etc.
- Don't leave doors and windows open, especially if the host doesn't know they have been opened.
- Never smoke inside without checking first.
- Ask before borrowing something and make sure you return items to your host before you leave.
- Never complain and remember to compliment your host – perhaps mention the cooking or the décor.
- Check before putting drinks down if coasters are needed.
- Always ask before using the phone or the internet.
- Make your bed each morning.
- Keep every room you use clean and tidy and don't leave your belongings out.
- Don't leave food, glasses or cups in your bedroom.
- Keep your bathroom clean and use the towels sparingly.
- If sharing a bathroom, carry your toiletries to and from the bathroom.
- Don't overstay your welcome!

The perfect hostess

Now we've talked about enjoying the hospitality of others with the best of manners, it's time to look at how to turn on the charm as a hostess. If there's one thing I could add to my CV, it's hotel management! Being a great hostess is all about being hospitable, about offering your home and your company to others with generosity. It's a good way to not only

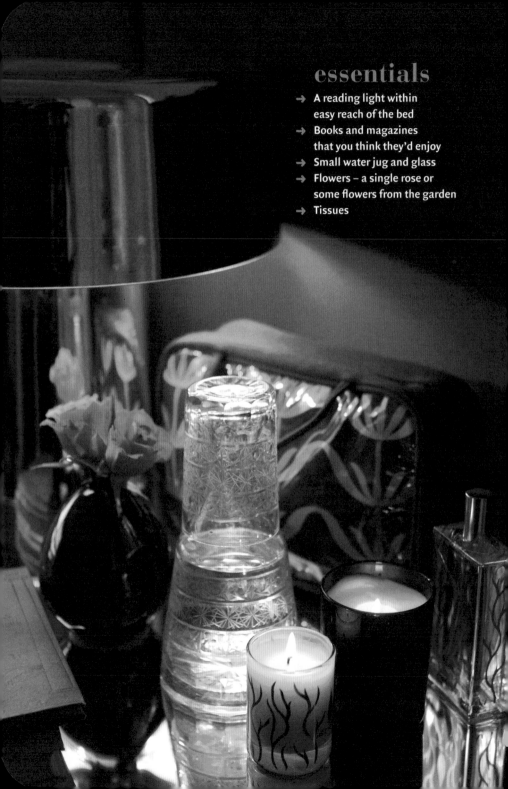

essentials

→ A reading light within
  easy reach of the bed
→ Books and magazines
  that you think they'd enjoy
→ Small water jug and glass
→ Flowers – a single rose or
  some flowers from the garden
→ Tissues

repay the kindness and hospitality of others, but also to get your friends together and have a great time. Entertaining others, or having guests to stay, should be fun. By being fully prepared and knowing what is expected, you will avoid a large amount of stress.

I find that the key to being a successful hostess is planning well in advance and being ultra-organised – the more I can do prior to the event, the better. I usually have a couple of contingency plans in case anything goes wrong – such as where you'll regroup from a picnic in the event of bad weather – and this way you'll be able to really relax and enjoy the event yourself. In this chapter we'll look across specific events such as dinner parties in detail, but we'll start off by going through the planning stages that will allow you to host a successful event.

Preparing a guest bedroom

Creating a cosy bedroom is one of the little treats you can offer any guests you have to stay. When visiting friends, it's always the small touches that mean a lot and leave a lasting impression on me. When you're preparing a guestroom, thinking ahead of everything your guest might need will add to the success of any visit, and it also makes your job as host more stress-free. Most importantly, having an attractive, fresh room for your guest makes them feel immediately welcome and comfortable in your home. Here are a few tips to think about – and also see opposite for a list of guestroom essentials.

- Make sure the room is thoroughly cleaned and aired before your guest arrives
- Check there are extra hangers for clothes and some drawer space
- Include clean folded towels
- Make up the bed with clean crisp sheets – fold an extra blanket at the end of the bed in case they get cold
- Make sure pillows are soft and comfy – and include both feathered and synthetic pillows in case of any allergies

Initial planning

As soon as you decide to host an event, whatever the occasion, it's a good idea to dig out your notebook and make a list of the ideas and details that first come into your head. You can then develop these ideas into more detailed checklists, shopping lists, worksheets and menu plans.

- First of all, consider how many guests you want to invite – if you're starting out, maybe begin with a small dinner party, and then hold a larger event once you're more confident in the role of hostess.
- Send invitations three to four weeks prior to your party and keep track of who can or can't attend, and if any guests have special dietary requirements.
- Think carefully about the menu – do you want to put on a full sit-down meal, drinks and nibbles, or a buffet? If you're cooking, keep it simple and make sure you're confident of the results. Do as much in advance of the day itself as possible.
- To be on the safe side, prepare extra vegetarian dishes – this also gives other guests an option if they happen not to like the main dish without drawing attention to themselves.
- Think about food presentation and what can be done to make each plate or buffet setting more attractive and presentable.
- If it's not a sit-down dinner, keep the party atmosphere going by constantly circulating small dishes and nibbles around the room.
- Consider specific design details depending on the event. For instance, think about table design, a colour scheme, if you have enough matching place mats, coasters, cutlery and crockery.
- Create the right atmosphere with lighting (lamps and candles), flowers (as a centrepiece or around the room) and background music (make sure it doesn't drown out conversation).
- Pay attention to small details – think about ashtrays, toothpicks, napkins, ice, after-dinner sweets and extra hand towels and toilet paper in the bathroom.

On the day

Although you've done as much planning and preparation as possible before the party, there are still a few things to remember on the day itself to make sure your event is hassle-free and runs as smoothly as possible. These following tips will help make your guests feel welcome, relaxed and in the mood for a good time.

- Create a schedule of timings so you know what you should be doing. You might not stick to it exactly, but it will give you a basic guide.
- If a friend offers to help out, then accept – an extra pair of hands is invaluable. This will relieve some of the pressure on you and give more time to spend with your guests.
- Always offer guests refreshments on arrival and keep an eye out for empty glasses later on.
- Have plenty of non-alcoholic options available, including water. Place water jugs and spare glasses around the room so guests can help themselves.
- Accept any gifts graciously.
- Make introductions and mention something interesting about your guests to encourage conversation, especially if people are meeting for the first time.
- Try to give your guests equal attention – some will be more demanding than others, so don't let them dominate your company!
- Try to keep conversations flowing and step in, if necessary, when awkward lulls occur. Be aware of anyone excluded from conversations and attempt to draw them in.
- Offer your guests second helpings of food, in case they are too embarrassed to ask.

As the hostess, you set the tone – if you're stressed, frantic and agitated, your guests may feel the same. Try to stay relaxed – you want to offer a warm, inviting and fun atmosphere. Most importantly, don't forget to join in the fun yourself – there's no point entertaining if you're the only person who doesn't enjoy themselves. I'm sure your friends would prefer to have the pleasure of your company and see you with a smile on your face rather than running around in a flap all night!

For detailed menu planners, worksheets and checklists that will help you entertain to perfection – head to www.lifestyle-essentials.com

Hosting a dinner party

A dinner party is one of my favourite ways to entertain and needn't be all that stressful – as long as you put in a bit of planning. I think it's lovely to gather your friends together in a welcoming environment with tasty food and good wine. It's also an opportunity to introduce friends who don't know each other and create different social dynamics.

All the tips and details we've already been through are useful for any type of event you host. For a dinner party, in addition to these, there are several more specific things that you should consider.

Receiving guests

The most important general rule to remember is that it's always far better to overestimate than underestimate the amount of food and drink you aim to serve!

- At a pre-dinner reception with drinks and appetisers, allow for five to seven appetisers per person per hour and roughly two drinks per person per hour (wine and champagne bottles have around five to six servings, while a 750 ml bottle of spirits serves around sixteen highball, cocktail or mixed drinks).
- At dinner, allow half a bottle of wine per guest, and place red and white wine on the table along with bottles of still and sparkling water.
- Stock enough ice – allow half a pound to a pound per person.
- Have a good supply of glasses on hand – where possible, allowing guests to get a clean one at least twice during the night.

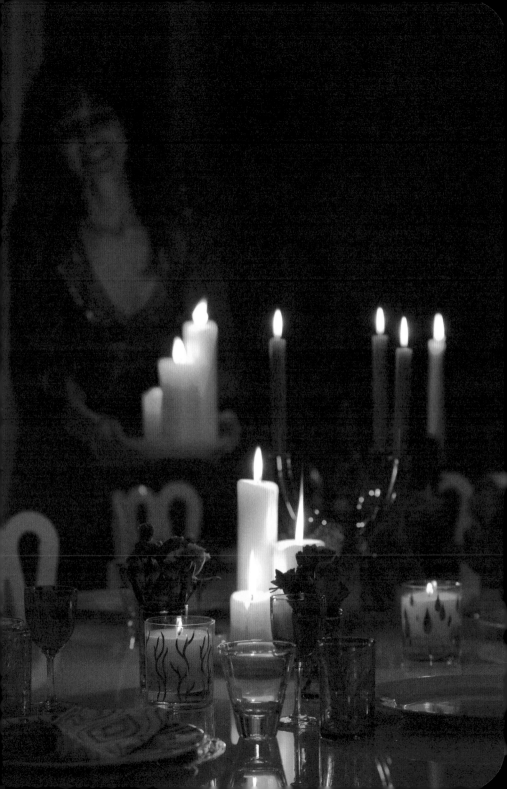

Setting a table

When preparing the table for dinner, give a little thought to presentation – it will make all the difference. If it's quite a formal affair you're hosting, here are some key tips to follow on laying the table.

- Create a symmetrical table by setting each place equidistant from the next, and centring them all around your table piece if you have one. Also make sure all guests will have enough elbow room.
- Start with a crisp and clean tablecloth – white or ivory are usually the best for a formal affair, but if you are having a specific colour theme, think carefully about which colours look good together. A dark tablecloth may make the table look smaller. If possible, use napkins in a matching colour or style to the tablecloth.
- Place the bottom of the silverware one inch from the edge of the table and arrange cutlery according to the order they will be used, working from the outside in.
- Place bread plates to the left of each setting, with glasses on the right.
- Place wine glasses outside of the water glasses.
- Place napkins as you prefer – folded, or using napkin rings, on top of the base plate or to the left of the forks.
- If you're using a seating arrangement, put seating cards above each plate, with the name facing the seat.

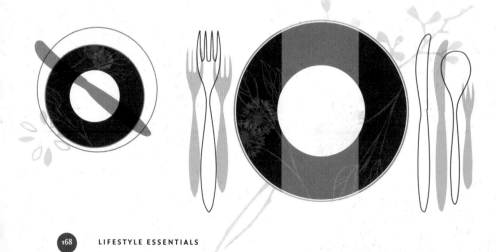

- Create a centrepiece, maybe using flowers or candles. Whatever the arrangement, make sure it's not too big, or it might obscure your guests' view of each other.
- Light any candles at least five minutes before guests enter the room.
- Place enough salt and pepper mills and butter dishes on the table – a group of eight people needs two sets of each.
- Use glass jars or bowls with small serving spoons for any condiments such as sauce or horseradish.
- Make sure there's enough water on your table – put bottles or pitchers of still and sparkling water at each end of the table.
- For an extra touch, use decorative bowls in empty spaces and fill them with sweets and after-dinner treats.

Seating guests

It's actually far harder than it might seem to create a successful seating plan. You need to be aware of your guests' personalities and interests to make sure those sitting next to each other have plenty to talk about and won't clash. These tips below might help.

- I always start by placing my husband and myself on either side of the table (directly opposite each other) and then work my way round from there.
- Write the name of each guest on a Post-it note to play around with seating options until you've made a decision.
- If possible, try to seat men and women next to each other, so it goes: boy, girl, boy, girl and so on, around the table.
- Consider placing yourself closest to the kitchen so you don't disrupt other guests when moving back and forth.
- As a general rule, separate partners from each other – they see each other all the time anyway! Meeting new people and discussing different topics make dinner parties more interesting. Although you might decide to place guests who don't know anyone else, or who struggle with social interaction, next to their partners.

- Be creative and adventurous – it can be fun! Through clever seating plans you might create new friendships, or even play matchmaker!
- If you'll be getting up from your seat a lot throughout dinner, place understanding and confident guests either side of you.
- If the seating plan doesn't seem to be working out on the night, suggest switching places after the main meal. According to tradition, you might ask ladies to remain still while the men move round a certain number of places.

Serving food

When it comes to serving your food, there's a whole host of things to think about – so here are a few helpful pointers.

- Put out pre-dinner nibbles for guests to snack on, just in case you're running late with dinner.
- Never use paper plates or disposable cutlery, unless you are hosting a barbecue or a children's party. Try to use matching sets of china and cutlery where possible – if it's an extra special event and you don't have enough, consider borrowing from a friend or hiring enough for the evening.
- If there's room, use a serving table or sideboard so you don't have to keep running between table and kitchen. Use it for hotplates to keep food warm and for serving utensils and extra cutlery.
- If there's room on the dining table, set out cold courses such as salad before the guests arrive. But keep cheese platters away from the table until the rest of the meal has been finished.
- Water glasses can be filled beforehand, but wine should not be served until guests are seated at the table. If offering both red and white wine, offer the white first.
- If you want your meal to be very formal, serve food according to the traditional order of female guests first, eldest to youngest, leaving yourself until last. Then serve males, eldest to youngest. Clear food away in the same order.

- Always serve food on the left side of the person, which is the fork side. I remember this by thinking food and fork both start with 'F'. Always clear from the right.
- Serve beverages on the right, which is the same side as the glasses.
- If serving a roast, for instance, you can serve meat on each plate but allow guests to serve vegetables and side dishes themselves.
- For large dinners or lunches, consider serving food as a buffet and let guests help themselves. If you choose this option, keep food hot using chafing dishes or hotplates.
- For a buffet served on a freestanding rectangular table, place the stack of plates at the start of the queue, then place food dishes in a sensible order as they'd be served – generally: main dish, side dishes, accompaniments, sauces, bread and then cutlery. Napkins can be stacked between the plates or wrapped around the cutlery. Mirror the arrangement of dishes, so you can have two lines of guests serving themselves at the same time.
- With a buffet, place drinks and glasses on a separate table, and also serve dessert, tea and coffee from a different table.

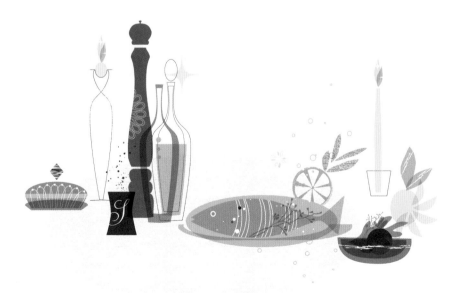

Hosting a cocktail party

Cocktail parties have become more popular than ever – they're a simple yet effective way to entertain your friends or colleagues or to have a special girls' night in!

For obvious reasons, a cocktail party can be a lot of fun, and is also an easier alternative to a full-blown dinner party – there's much less preparation and tidying up involved. Once you've thrown together a few delicious, exotic drinks, along with some great finger foods, you're pretty much done – and the main focus of the night rests on mingling and catching up.

Cocktail parties can be glamorously sophisticated or casual and informal – it's entirely up to you. But what better excuse to throw on that fabulously sexy cocktail dress you've been keeping hidden in your wardrobe!

Party checklist

- Send out handwritten invites to your chosen guests – cocktail parties usually start between 6.30 and 8.30 pm and last for two to three hours.
- Get hold of a cocktail recipe book so you know how to mix a variety of options. It's worth experimenting a few times before the party if you are mixing any cocktails for the first time – get a couple of friends over and try them out together!
- If you're inviting a large number of guests or hosting a very formal cocktail party, consider hiring a bartender. This frees up more time for you to mingle and be sociable and is also likely to increase the variety and adventurousness of drinks you are serving.
- Make sure your bar's well-stocked, and that you have an assortment of glasses, depending on the drinks you'll be serving, and a variety of mixers – including orange juice, soda, tonic, ginger ale, Coca-Cola, tomato juice, Tabasco sauce, lemons, limes, horseradish, and Worcestershire sauce.

- Decorate your home with flowers and create a party atmosphere with scented candles and party lights – make sure it's not too dark though, as people want to mingle and chat.
- Allocate an area for coats – perhaps by clearing a hallway closet.
- Make sure you have enough extra seating for the party.
- Get together some great lounge music compilations.
- Have coffee available for any guests who want to wake up a little before heading home (although remember that drinking coffee does not help you to sober up).
- Have the telephone number of local taxi companies at hand for guests who aren't driving home.

The drinks

Cocktails are delightful, playful drinks, especially when drunk from the appropriate glasses. Cosmopolitans, Martinis, Mojitos, Caipirinhas and Peach Bellinis are all really delicious and my absolute favourites. Make sure you don't forget about those who might not drink alcohol. Always have plenty of water and the usual soft-drink options on stand-by, but why not also serve a great non-alcoholic cocktail – this'll stop your non-drinking guests from feeling left out of all the fun.

My website includes my favourite cocktail recipes – just head to www.lifestyle-essentials.com

essentials

- → Cocktail shaker
- → Electric blender
- → Juicer
- → Strainer
- → Jigger (measuring device)
- → Bottle opener and corkscrew
- → Cutting board
- → Grater
- → Ice bucket
- → Tongs
- → Stirrers
- → Plenty of ice (about a pound of ice per guest)
- → A variety of garnishes – olives, cherries, etc ...
- → Cocktail napkins

Party food

The great thing about cocktail party food is that it can be a fun, eclectic selection of items and you can make just about anything you want. When estimating food quantities, cater for around five to seven bites per person per hour. Here is a selection of my favourite tasty treats.

Savoury canapés	Vegetarian canapés	Sweet canapés
Cocktail sausage baked in honey and mustard	Cheese stuffed mushrooms	Baby chocolate éclairs
Smoked salmon on sliced buttered bread, cut into triangles	Small vegetable spring rolls	Fresh-cut fruit on skewers
Filo-wrapped prawns	Vegetable tempura with soy sauce	Mini cupcakes
Grilled prawns on skewers	Vegetarian sushi	Chocolate-covered strawberries
Boiled new potatoes sliced in half, topped with crème fraiche and caviar.	Haloumi, sun-blushed tomato and olive skewers	Mini meringues with kiwi and passionfruit on top
Chicken satay on skewers	Feta and spinach filo triangles	Strawberry shortbreads
Small spring rolls – pork or beef	Mini risotto balls	Selection of baklava

Tasty nibbles

Make sure you keep nibbles on hand for when guests arrive unexpectedly. Whatever the occasion, when guests come over, it is considered thoughtful and hospitable to put out some small bowls of nibbles on a tray; for some simple yet satisfying ideas, see opposite.

essentials

→ Vegetable sticks – carrots, red, yellow and green peppers, cucumber, etc – around a bowl of sour-cream-and chive dip or some hummus
→ Crisps
→ Olives
→ Pistachio nuts
→ Cheesy sticks and breadsticks

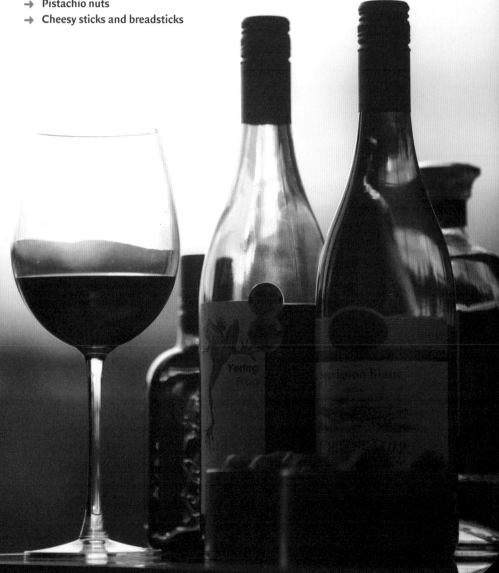

Girls' night in

Having some fun, catch-up time with your girlfriends is extremely important, and you don't need to hit the town to do it either. Why not invite over your close girlfriends and host a girls' night in? Choose one or two yummy cocktails you can mix up together, put out some nibbles and perhaps order some gourmet pizzas. You can load up your iPod with some groovy tunes and play a game while gossiping. My favourite games are charades, gin rummy (the card game), and Boggle! For something really different, you could organise a regular dance class in your house, like salsa. Or to indulge your tastebuds, host an exotic food-tasting evening where each person brings a new dish, or a monthly cooking class.

Time for tea

When you want to impress a guest or charm your friends, and a bowl of crisps just won't cut it – you know it's time for tea. I also love to invite guests for the weekend to arrive at tea time – it makes a lovely welcome, especially in winter when it's miserable outside. The other fantastic thing about tea is that you can serve it for any number of people – from an intimate catch-up between two people, to a formal tea party for 50!

An afternoon tea usually starts between 3 and 5 pm. The tradition is believed to have begun with Anna, Duchess of Bedford in the early 19th century – she'd order a pot of tea and snacks to stave off mid-afternoon hunger pangs before the evening meal.

While the food can be quite simple to prepare, there's also plenty of room for creativity at tea time. I love serving up all kinds of fun and delicious goodies – an array of savoury and sweet treats that you can hold between your finger and thumb.

Teatime treats

At teatime, I always serve food on a three-tiered cake tray – with sandwiches on the bottom, scones, cupcakes or sliced cake in the middle, and sweet tidbits on top – think biscuits, chocolate truffles, nougat and Turkish delight! At a formal tea party – if the food is laid out on the table, you should start with the scones or cake, then try the tiny sandwiches, before finishing off with the sweets. Think of it like a meal, where you have bread first, then the main course and save the dessert for last.

Traditional tea sandwiches are usually small (a regular-size sandwich cut into four squares, four triangles, or about three fingers), made from thinly sliced bread, and have their crusts cut off. Spread each one with butter or cream cheese, and then choose from a variety of fillings.

Traditional fillings include cucumber, cheese and tomato, egg salad and smoked salmon with cream cheese, but you don't have to keep them plain! These days you can add garlic, mustard, pepper, sauces and any type of filling you like.

essentials

- → large tray
- → two teapots (one for English Breakfast and the other for Earl Grey)
- → small jug of milk
- → bowl of sugar with spoon (or serve sugar lumps with tongs)
- → honey
- → dish of lemon slices with small fork
- → teacups, saucers and teaspoons
- → small plates, knives and forks
- → cocktail napkins
- → tiered cake tray with selection of sweet and savoury food

The art of gift giving

One of the greatest joys of life is giving presents to others – and seeing their surprise and enthusiasm when they receive them. And topping this enjoyment is giving someone a personal gift that they will really value. There's a special charm in a present that can't just be bought in any old shop – something unique, well thought out or even handmade. These are truly the best gifts – especially for people who already have or can afford to buy anything they want.

Remember – there are plenty of other opportunities to give gifts besides birthdays and Christmas. You can give one to celebrate a special occasion or achievement, to a friend who needs cheering up, or to say thank you for any number of reasons. It will create a warm glow for the two of you.

tips

→ Create a gift ideas list so you're never short of ideas. Do your homework and ask people for hints or a wish list.

→ The amount you spend on a gift should be a balance of your affection for that person combined with what your budget will allow.

→ Look while doing normal shopping or shopping in the sales – you get great bargains that way and won't be rushed into any inappropriate last-minute gift purchases.

→ Browse for gifts on websites as well – take up free shipping opportunities.

→ Make gifts personal by engraving or monogramming gifts.

→ Send friends or family who live abroad gifts which remind them of back home or vice versa – send gifts distinctive to another culture.

→ If you take care in selecting a gift, also take care in wrapping it. Put gifts in boxes before wrapping – either from the store it came from, or in an unmarked or decorative box. If using a gift bag, wrap the present in tissue paper. Decorate a plain gift bag or wrapping with ribbon, glitter or stars to make it extra special.

→ Complete the gift with a handwritten card of well wishes and love – the more personal the message the better.

'The excellence of a gift lies in its appropriateness rather than in its value.' Charles Dudley Warner

The art of regifting

How many of us receive gifts that aren't suitable or to our taste, that don't fit or are just plain not right, and that you know you will never use? It happens to all of us from time to time, and when it does, you've got two options. You can stick the unwanted present in a cupboard never to be seen again, or you could give it to someone else.

However, regifting does require some thought. Gifts should only be recycled when you're certain that the recipient would really like to receive it; that the gift is brand new and comes with its original packaging; and that the original giver didn't take great care to select it especially just for you. And if you're concerned that a friend might be offended by receiving a recycled gift, don't pass it on – it's not worth damaging a friendship over.

tips

→ Start a gift cupboard – I stash all my recyclers in it. Although a gift's not to your taste, it may be to someone else's. Hold on to it until the right opportunity comes up to pass the gift on.

→ Make sure you don't get caught regifting – you wouldn't want to offend the person who gave you the gift in the first place. Keep a list of the gifts you intend to regift and who gave them to you.

→ If you're regifting a gift that's been stored away for months, make sure it's in perfect condition first.

→ Regift to charity – wrap them up again with fresh wrapping paper and take them to a children's hospital, a nursing home or a homeless shelter, where they'll be greatly appreciated.

→ Offer them as raffle prizes for charity fundraisers.

→ Mix a recycled gift with a new gift – no guilt and double the gift!

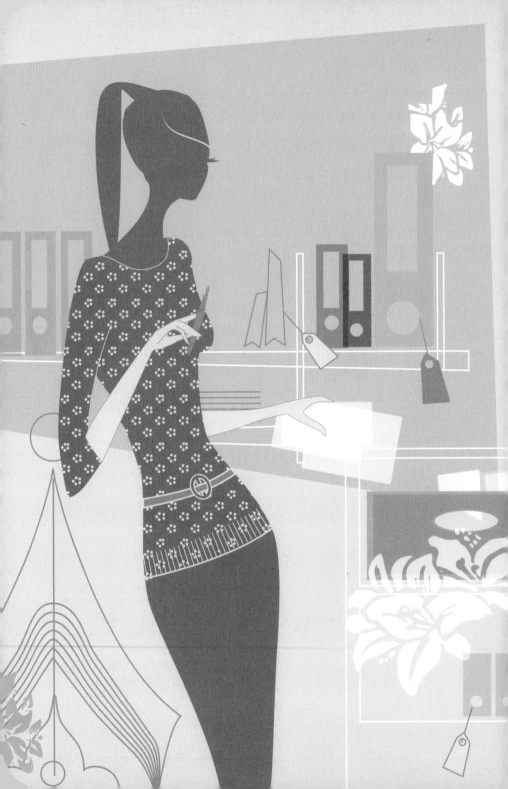

7
the organised you

I firmly believe that if you're organised in your personal life, it will have a positive influence on all other aspects of your life, helping you to achieve and enjoy a fulfilled lifestyle.

Time is a valuable commodity – there never seems to be enough of it in the day to fit everything in. So how can you successfully juggle work, family, hobbies, your social life and your personal time and still enjoy life to the fullest? By learning how to organise your time, you can keep everything running smoothly and generally feel you have achieved the most you can. In my opinion, good time management is crucial – as it leaves you more successful, satisfied, efficient, productive and relaxed about life in general. It also gives you more time for the parts of life that you really enjoy!

'Out of clutter, find Simplicity. From discord, find Harmony. In the middle of difficulty lies opportunity.'
Albert Einstein

How to get organised

So, what can you do to get yourself organised? Let's start by looking at some general techniques to keep basic routines under control. We can then look more closely at specific parts of life that need more organising than others, such as your house and your holidays.

Time management

Being organised is actually about simplifying life but it takes self-discipline to make decisions and stick to them. To manage time efficiently you need to stay focused and determined. Prioritise the things you need to achieve and allocate a suitable amount of time to each. Set yourself goals, keep the end results in mind and put care and thought into your actions.

Admin management

Ever noticed how, for every project you're working on, you accumulate piles of paperwork, notes, letters and endless bits and pieces? If you find that these are always getting mixed up or lost – then you need to work out ways of improving your current admin system, or create one from scratch!

I find the simplest way of handling admin is to create a project binder – either one for each project or one large binder containing notes for all current jobs. Keep all paperwork together using subject dividers and plastic pockets and add an index if you have lots of information. Put a date reference on anything you file and make sure sections are clearly marked. Having all the information you need at your fingertips will save a lot of time and makes life much easier.

When documents come in that aren't part of a current project, you should discard or file them away immediately.

Create systems and routines

A simple, yet very effective way of staying organised is to implement systems or routines – and stick to them! Systems, checklists and worksheets allow you to manage your time more efficiently. They jog your memory when something needs to be done, and we all know how fulfilling it is to cross things off as we complete them! These are the tools I find most useful in managing my time.

Personal 'To Do' list – I make a daily list of everything I need to get done and tick tasks off as I achieve them.

Calendar – Rather than using a diary, I create and update my calendar using Outlook on my computer, which also synchs with my Blackberry. I use this to keep on top of activities, birthdays, anniversaries, special events, holidays and anything else I need to remember. It includes times, venues and any contact details so all information is in the one place. I then print an A4 page of each month and keep one copy in my handbag and the other on the bulletin board in my kitchen, so all the household can see it. If you don't have Outlook, you can download a monthly calendar worksheet from www.lifestyle-essentials.com.

Personal categorised contacts list – I keep one central list of the details of my contacts, whether family, friends or work colleagues – including their addresses, telephone numbers and emails. I add anyone I might need in a hurry, such as my doctor, dentist, school contacts, emergency services and local council details. It's much easier having them all together rather than having to search through several address books and pieces of paper.

You can go to my website for all kinds of templates for useful checklists and worksheets – www.lifestyle-essentials.com

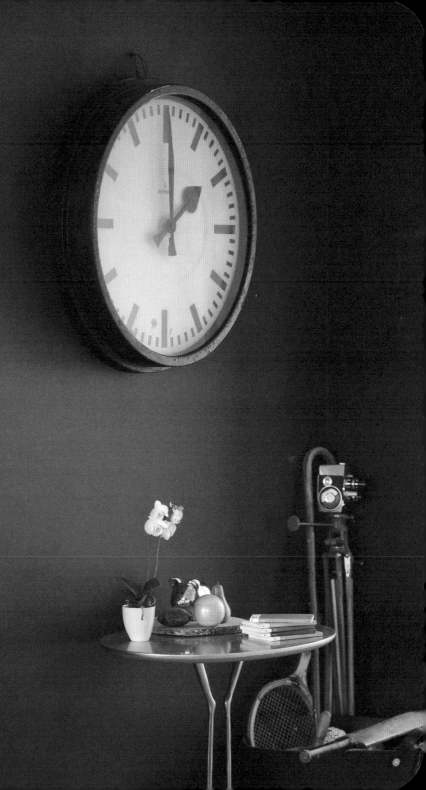

Lisa's To Do List

Things to do

- [ ] Upload photo images from weekend to be printed
- [ ] Book flights to Florida
- [ ] Diarise with Anton

Things to get

- [ ] Flowers for house
- [ ] Satinwood paint for new radiator covers
- [ ] Birthday present for Uncle Laurie
- [ ] Picture frame for new photo of Orlando & Noah for Daddy's office

Errands to run

- [ ] Supermarket – need rice milk, peanut butter & bread
- [ ] Pharmacy – Get passport photo taken for new passport
- [ ] Post office – post passport renewal form along with expired passport
- [ ] Dry cleaners – pick up winter coats

Bills to pay

- [ ] Gym membership
- [ ] M&S card
- [ ] 123 Reg – domain name renewal
- [ ] Orlando's swimming class

Calls to make

- [ ] Call Mum to let her know dates I can visit
- [ ] Karen at Models One re fashion show for NSPCC
- [ ] Linda to arrange playdate for kids
- [ ] Helen at Crave Maternity to discuss photoshoot for Lifestyle Essentials
- [ ] Book appointment with dental hygienist

Appointments

- [ ] 11 am – take Noah to clinic for his MMR shots
- [ ] 1 pm – hair appointment at Daniel Hersheson's
- [ ] 4 pm – meeting with Robin to discuss progress of mothers4children.org

More things to remember

- [ ] Practise song with Orlando for his school play – he needs all-white clothing too
- [ ] Find fabric for curtains in the guest bedroom
- [ ] Need to get new stationery printed soon – running low!

Personal statistics and information

Another organisational tip is keeping a record of your personal statistics at hand. You never know when you might need to fill out an insurance or medical form, or some other important document. This record can also be very useful when travelling – do you actually know all of your stats in both metric and imperial? It could also be useful to know your vital statistics and clothes sizes for future shopping sprees – make sure you know the conversions from UK to both European and US sizes!

At the least, make note of the following information – head to www.lifestyle-essentials.com for easy-to-use templates and PDFs.

my statistics

NAME:

DATE OF BIRTH:

WEIGHT:

BLOOD TYPE:

WAIST MEASUREMENT:

ALLERGIES:

BUST MEASUREMENT:

MEDICATION:

INNER LEG MEASUREMENT:

DOCTOR'S DETAILS:

SHOE SIZE:

HEIGHT:

DRESS SIZE:

Household organisation

In the next chapter, I talk more about the role of your home in creating a balanced life for yourself, so for now I'll just emphasise how important it is to come home at the end of the day to a house that is organised, comfortable and suits the way you live.

The basic upkeep of your home is not exactly fun but it has to be done, even though there are so many other things you'd rather be doing. By using basic organisational skills you can run your home smoothly and have plenty of time left over for all of the other things in life. With two kids, an energy-filled entrepreneurial husband, two homes, work commitments, charity work, friends, family and dogs, it took me a while to learn to balance opposing pressures, but I now know how to run my household efficiently to keep everyone happy – and have even become known as the Chief of Stuff!

Let's look at a few ways you can get organised to make running your household easier on yourself.

Create a household binder

I find my household binder priceless – creating one is the ideal way to keep together all of the essential information you need for good household management at your fingertips.

My household binder is not only very useful for me but also for my partner and for babysitters. It keeps them informed about details they might need to know and gives them an idea of how to react in various situations. This, in turn, keeps the house running smoothly and creates a stable and reliable environment.

The following list shows some of the items you might need in your master binder for quick access. Go to my website to download the readymade templates.

Contacts

Keep important contact details for your doctor, dentist, optometrist, emergency surgery, nearest pharmacy, emergency services and local police station. It's also important to include a list of contractors and suppliers for your house, such as an electrician, plumber, window cleaner and so on.

Emergencies

Keep a note of what to do and who to contact in an emergency. In addition to the contact details above, work out what you would do if something was to go wrong with the house, and how you would handle it. For example, make note of all fire alarms and ensure they're checked regularly. List all exits and any alternative ways of leaving the house in case of a fire. Similarly, know where your water mains shut off valves are in case there's a leak or flooding, and note where the circuit breaker switches are in case of a power cut. This might also be a good time to make sure you have plenty of spare candles, matches, torches, batteries and other emergency supplies and store them in an easily accessible place.

Household utilities

Keep a list of all your main utility suppliers and service providers. These include gas, electricity, water, council tax, telephone, broadband and television. Note account numbers and reference numbers for each, and how you pay for each – direct debit, cheques etc. This information will help make any queries you have much easier to sort out. Also, make sure you know where meters are and how to read them yourself. This way you can double-check the bills as they come in.

Home maintenance

You should record any home maintenance or repairs in the same way you record your own medical history. If something breaks down suddenly, it's incredibly useful to know when it was last checked or repaired, by whom and what work was done. Also keep track of any cosmetic work, building work and decorating that's carried out on your house.

Household appliances

If you can, keep all paperwork from household appliances, including warranty details and the dates and places of purchase. These might mean that you get repairs carried out free of charge, if still in date. Also hang on to your manuals. I always used to throw them away once I had something up and running, but if something goes wrong, having instructions can actually be a big help.

Household inventories

A home inventory is a complete and detailed list of all the personal property located in your home. It takes time to do an inventory, but it's useful for insurance purposes in the event of fire or theft and also helps keep track of your material worth. Take each room one at a time and list all contents. Be as detailed as possible, including serial numbers and

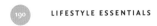

descriptions where appropriate, and an estimate of the purchase price if you don't have the receipt. It's also a good idea to keep a copy of the inventory, in a safe place, outside your home.

Family favourites

Aside from all the serious stuff, your household binder can also include more fun information, such as favourite recipes or restaurant contact details.

Private and confidential

There are certain private details that you should keep together, but which are just for your own reference. Rather than keeping these in the household binder, make a personal file for yourself, and then keep the originals in a secure place for safety.

- Banking and credit card details
- Financial investments
- Legal documents
- Mortgage documents or rental agreements
- Insurance documents
- Marriage certificate
- Birth certificates
- Will
- Passport
- Driving licence

Add any other information you need to these items – for instance, contact details for your bank manager, solicitor or financial advisor. Also make note of any actions required to keep these documents current – such as renewing insurance policies or your passport.

You might find it useful to record everything on a summary sheet so you have all the details you need on one piece of paper for easy reference.

For my ideas, visit www.lifestyle-essentials.com

Your car

One thing my brother has taught me well is that if you want to get the most out of your car, you need to look after it properly. A well-maintained vehicle runs more efficiently, is safer, kinder on the environment, and lasts longer. With this in mind, you need to be organised when running a car, both to reduce the risk of breaking down and so you don't get hit with huge repair bills or fines.

To take care of your car, some basic car maintenance knowledge is essential and will also save you money in the long run. If in doubt, consult your car manual, or ask someone in the know (either a mechanic, friend or partner) to show you how to carry out the following checks so you can do them yourself in future.

Car checks

Tyres – Check the treads on your tyres are not worn or uneven (there's a legal minimum tread depth and it's dangerous to drive with poor tread). Check the tyre pressure, based on the recommended pressure figures given in your owner's manual – it's common for different amounts to be recommended for the front and back tyres. Most garages have a user-friendly air hose, which you can use to top up your tyres to the correct level – it's much easier than you'd think to do this yourself.

Engine oil level – Check your engine oil levels using the dipstick that usually protrudes from the side of the engine. Pull it out and wipe it clean before inserting it back. When you pull it out again the oil mark should be between the upper and lower limit markings on the dipstick. If you need to top up the oil, check which type of oil you require in your manual – petrol stations should carry all types.

LIFESTYLE ESSENTIALS

Windscreen washer fluid – Check your washer fluid levels and top up if required. Some screen wash is concentrated, so you need to dilute it with water to the ratio listed on the bottle.

Brakes – Check your handbrake by parking on a hill. Pull up the brake and if it takes more than a few clicks before holding on the hill, you need to get it looked at by a professional mechanic. Keep an eye out for brake fluid leaking under the pedal on the floor or carpet and be aware of changes in your brake pedal movement based on when your brakes begin to bite. If you notice significant changes, have them checked by a mechanic.

Lights – Keep an eye out to make sure your brakelights, headlights, tail-lights and indicator lights are all working. If you notice a light is not working, you might simply need to change the bulb, and these can be purchased cheaply at any auto parts shop.

Services

It's very important to have your car regularly serviced – a qualified mechanic runs a series of checks to ensure the car is safe and reliable to drive and picks up on any potential problems. The regularity and content of a service depends on the model, age and mileage of your car.

You should always ask for a service history logbook when purchasing a car, as this will show past services and checks. It also gives you recommendations for when you should carry out a service – usually after a certain number of miles or length of time (whichever happens first). The more miles you drive, the more frequently you should service your car.

Make sure the mechanic stamps your logbook at each service, including the date and mileage. This way you can keep on top of when your car needs its next service – but it's also important if you intend to resell your car, as a full service history is often requested.

MOT

All vehicles need to comply with minimum road safety and environmental standards, so if you have a vehicle older than three years, you need to have an MOT (Ministry of Transport) test with a qualified tester once a year. You also need a valid MOT certificate to purchase car insurance and to renew your car tax, so don't forget to book your car in every year.

How to keep track

To keep track of checks, services and MOT dates, it's a good idea to create an information sheet for your car, in addition to keeping your logbook updated. There's a template on my website including the details listed in checklist 1. Go to www.lifestyle-essentials.com.

Keep a copy in your glovebox so you have all the information you need in case of an emergency or when speaking to a mechanic. Also add reminders to your calendar or diary so you don't forget to book your car in for its next service or MOT.

Be prepared

Finally, I always try to be prepared for any eventuality. If you're like me, keep a few items of emergency equipment in the car, like those in the second checklist.

checklist

→ registration number
→ make and model
→ engine size
→ number of doors
→ dates of services
→ dates of MOTs
→ insurance company and policy details
→ emergency recovery and breakdown information
→ repairs or maintenance

1

checklist

→ spare tyre
→ tyre-changing tools
→ jumpleads
→ petrol canister
→ emergency breakdown reflectors
→ first aid kit
→ spare blanket
→ bottle of water
→ energy snacks
→ torch
→ roadmap
→ pen and pad
→ spare change
→ tissues and handwipes
→ phone charger
→ disposable camera (to document any accident or incident)

2

The professional you

For many of us, our professional careers are a part of how we measure our personal success – and can be one of the key areas of our lives that we want to develop and continue to set goals for. In order to get the most out of your careers, it really helps to stay organised and focused – there are several things you can do, even if you're not actively looking to change jobs, that may make a difference to your future prospects.

You can continually be thinking about ways that you can gain new experience and knowledge that might benefit you – whether through a specific course or conference, or by attending networking events. Your employer may well be happy to pay for training directly relevant to your job, so ask to see what extra training is available to you. If not, paying for yourself can still be a worthwhile investment – taking initiative can often be the pivotal factor that helps you to get that promotion or move to a new job that interests you more.

It also pays to keep your CV up to date – make sure you keep a detailed record of your employment history, contact details of referees, and all other relevant information – such as training courses. This makes it much easier to take the step to apply for new jobs, as it doesn't seem like such a massive chore to get your CV in order. Or say, for instance, you meet somebody and get chatting about your experience and they suddenly announce they know of the perfect opportunity for you ... if you can only email through your CV that afternoon. OK, it's a dream scenario, but stranger things have happened. Being prepared means you're ready to go and won't miss out!

Decide what you really want

I believe it's crucial to feel happy with your career. Life's too short to spend so much of your time doing something you don't enjoy or feel passionate about. The more you enjoy your job, the more enthusiasm and dedication you will invest into it. You'll be more likely to be good at what you do and will feel more fulfilled with life overall. So it's worth bearing this in mind when assessing your current career or considering taking a new direction – and an organised approach will help you make the best career decisions for yourself.

As I'm more of an artistic spirit myself – someone who enjoys creating and performing – this led me to pursue several careers in entertainment and fashion simultaneously. It suits my nature to have the freedom to move between different fields as and when opportunities arise.

Do a little soul-searching to determine what interests, inspires and motivates you – the kind of job that will give you back energy as well as taking it. Try writing down what appeals to you – regardless of education, skills and monetary requirements. Identify your likes and dislikes, analyse your strengths and weaknesses, and look at where you are in your professional life compared with where you'd like to be. Here are some active steps you can take towards achieving what you want.

Set time-restricted goals – Look at your time and ask how you're using it. Are you doing things that move you in the direction of your dreams?

Research – Learn everything you can about the careers or jobs that appeal to you, including what new skills you'd need and whether they're realistically achievable. Knowledge is key, so gather together all the information you can.

Listen and learn – Talk to people who work in a field that interests you. Find out the best and worst parts of the job. Ask them what they did to get to where they are, and what advice they can pass on to you.

Talk the talk – Networking is an essential part of any business success, so use any connections you have and make the most of any networking opportunities. Talk to people about what you want to do – you never know who may have valuable contacts or useful input. Collect business cards and create a business contacts database – write notes on the back of the cards to remind you of who the person is, where you met them and how they might be helpful to your career.

Try it on for size – If you're starting out, or switching career completely, see if you can test out your dream job by doing work experience. Make sure you enjoy it before deciding it's what you really want to do.

Once you've identified what you want to do, don't be deterred by any obstacles and challenges. Face them head-on, set yourself goals, and – most importantly – be positive!

Your CV – how to impress

We've already talked about the importance of first impressions when you meet somebody. In the professional world, your CV does this job for you – it's your introduction to a potential employer, so you want it to be as close to perfect as possible, meaning it's presented cleanly and clearly and shows off your qualifications and ability to do the job. When competition for a certain job is intense, there's no room for error on your CV, and even small slips can let you down. On the next page are a few CV dos and don'ts to help increase your chances at scoring that ideal job.

Go to my website for a whole bunch of useful templates – both for your CV and for career worksheets, which you can then customise for yourself: www.lifestyle-essentials.com

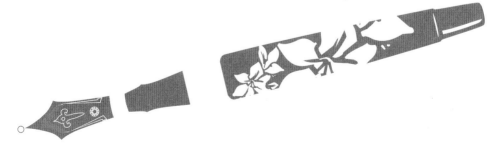

DO

→ keep it to a maximum of two typed pages – concentrate on quality of information, not quantity

→ consider your layout – make sure headings are accurate and stand out, use short and brief bullet point lists; key areas need to be clear and easily understood

→ use the spelling and grammar check on your computer to look for errors, but don't rely on this alone

→ ask someone else to check your CV for errors – there'll almost always be something you've missed

→ print your CV on good quality A4 paper in white or ivory

→ keep a complete list of your achievements and professional development separately – you can then tailor your CV to the specific job or company

→ customise your CV for each job/ company so that it's as relevant as it can be

→ send a personalised cover letter with your CV which gives the context for how your work experience fits you for the job

→ reread your CV and cover letter before the interview – make sure you know what you've sent them!

DON'T

→ lie – it always comes out in the end … if in doubt, leave it out!

→ decorate your CV – keep it free of borders, clip art, patterns, extravagant fonts and all other unnecessary embellishments

→ include personal details such as age, height, weight, health conditions and photos – they're all unnecessary

→ list references on your CV – state that they're 'available upon request'. This way you'll know if a company is interested enough to contact them, and you can tell your referees to expect a call or email

→ use exact dates – months and years are enough

→ give reasons for a termination or leaving a job – it's better to explain these things in person

→ be negative about yourself – don't mention things you are bad at

'The closest one can get to perfection is on a resume.'

Anonymous

Preparing for interviews

So you've done all the legwork ... and now you've got an interview. You got the interview on the strength of your CV, so meeting the employer is your second chance to sell yourself – based purely on how you cope with the questions and the general impression you make – all within a relatively short amount of time.

With this in mind, here are some useful tips on how to get ahead in an interview.

- Be prepared – research both the company and the specific job to demonstrate enthusiasm, initiative and a genuine interest towards both.
- Think ahead – consider what questions they will ask you and make sure you can explain why you are a good fit for the job.
- Be presentable – your appearance can say, or at least imply, a lot about you, so dress appropriately (don't wear anything loud or revealing and avoid large gaudy jewellery). To feel your best, make sure your clothes are freshly cleaned and ironed.
- Promote a vibrant personality – be animated, dynamic and confident, but avoid any arrogance.
- Communicate well – speak clearly and concisely and make sure you can be easily heard.
- Maintain eye contact – look your interviewers in the eye when speaking or being spoken to. Avoid staring at the floor or looking around the room as this can imply nervousness or a lack of confidence.
- Make a positive last impression – when you finish your interview, thank the person for their time and leave with a smile.

Your finances

While looking after your finances can be a bore, unfortunately, there's no getting around the importance of this task. Whether your finances are healthy or a little bit under the weather, they obviously have an enormous impact on both the lifestyle you lead and your future. Having lots of money to spend can be fun in the short term, but doesn't contribute to your long-term happiness, while financial security definitely does. This means good financial management is crucial – managing your own budget, understanding how money can work for you and investing wisely. This will help you to put yourself in a very strong and secure position or improve the one you already enjoy – so it's time to get organised about it!

Income and expenditure

If your expenditure exceeds your income you will eventually find yourself in debt. Simple enough, it would seem – yet increasingly, women in the UK are finding themselves in debt. These days we're so used to always paying online or with credit cards that it's easy to ignore the reality of what's going on with our dosh.

Being aware of your income and expenditure levels is the first step to living within your means and staying worry- and debt-free. And the key to this is successful budgeting. You can then assess your expenditure and work out where you can save money.

Write a budget

To set yourself an accurate budget, you need to take a detailed look at what you currently earn and spend in a fixed period of time. If you haven't done it before, this exercise is usually a very eye-opening experience. You'll learn whether you're putting yourself further in debt each month or whether you have some extra money to spend or invest.

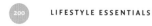

checklist

→ rent or mortgage
→ utilities – water, gas, electricity
→ telephone, broadband, mobile
→ TV licence, TV packages
→ council tax
→ insurance
→ pensions and investments
→ loan repayments
→ travel expenses
→ car expenses – insurance, tax, MOT, service and repairs, petrol
→ hair and beauty
→ groceries
→ clothes
→ toiletries and makeup
→ gym membership or fitness costs
→ hobbies
→ social – eating out, drinks, tickets, night clubs, taxis
→ holidays – travel/ flights, insurance, accommodation, meals, sightseeing
→ children – note all expenditure (this list doesn't end!)
→ pets

You can find a template for budgeting on my website – www.lifestyle-essentials.com – or just follow the steps below.

1 If you're paid monthly, use a month as your marker.

2 Write down your average monthly income after tax, based on your pay slip or bank statement.

3 Make a list of all your necessary expenditure in a month – see the list on the left.

4 Work out monthly averages for bills that you pay quarterly or yearly, or for amounts that vary from month to month.

5 Look at everything extra that you spend – be honest with yourself and use receipts and invoices where possible to find exact amounts.

6 Add up your total monthly expenditure.

7 If you have a joint income and share expenses, then include your partner's income figure and expenditure to your total amounts.

8 Subtract your total expenditure figure from your income.

If you have a healthy positive figure at the end, then obviously you're living within your means. If you have a negative or a low or break-even figure, your best bet is to review your expenditure list and see how you can change your spending habits and adjust your lifestyle.

Time to cut back?

If you simply spend too much, take a long hard look at your list and start prioritising to work out what you can live without. Be strict with yourself and cut back on non-essential extras. Set yourself an expenditure limit for each of these extras and stick to it – it's time to stop flashing your plastic.

Work towards clear goals with the money you save, such as paying off debt each month, or putting a certain amount aside to be invested. Use savings incentives, such as setting up an ISA (explained on p.204) and using a proportion of what you save for holidays or other extravagances.

What NOT to do ...
1 use a pawnbroker
2 take out a loan to pay off your debt
3 use credit cards and store cards to pay for items
4 borrow from a friend

My friends often joke that the B in my name stands for Lisa Bargain-Hunter. In his speech at my wedding, my husband's brother even made a gag about my habits, teasing: 'She saves it ... He spends it!' I guess the saying 'you can take the girl out of Brooklyn, but you can't take the Brooklyn out of the girl' is pretty accurate about me. Here are some of my top tips for saving – there are lots of ways to save, and they don't take a lot of effort, just a little bit of thought.

Top saving tips
● Wait for the sales to buy anything and everything
● If you find an incredible bargain, buy several and stash them away for gifts
● Buy in bulk (I particularly love Costco for this – an American cash-and-carry warehouse which has finally made it to England)

- Collect points religiously for every store (and do the same on flights – I've even managed to fly my family to visit me for free)
- Sign your utility accounts on to whatever points systems are offered, and arrange for direct debits too, as these often save you money
- Shop online – once you're a member you get sent special offers and discounts, and often get free shipping (which saves you time and the cost of your own transport). Online retailers also often offer more competitive prices because they don't pay overheads
- Don't pay interest on anything – make sure you budget so you can pay all of your credit card and utility bills as soon as you get them, and avoid late payment charges and interest fees. I can't bear the thought of wasting money in this way!

Savings and investments

While it's very easy to live for the moment, it's also important to consider your future. If you're successfully managing your budget and have money to spare each month, then investigate what savings and investment options are available to you. Even if you're struggling to live within your means, try incorporating at least a small amount for savings into your budget.

By saving, you may have a set goal in mind or just be giving yourself a bit of a buffer for life's unexpected curveballs. Maybe you want to go travelling for a few months or need a deposit for a house – whatever it's for, the money will definitely be appreciated at some point when you want to avoid borrowing.

These days there are endless savings options available to you – all with a variety of terms and conditions. In general, savings accounts keep your money safe and allow you to get to it fairly easily. At the end of the day, you get back whatever you put in, plus whatever interest you earn (although you are usually taxed on this interest).

Here's a quick guide to types of savings accounts – for more detailed information visit local branches of banks and building societies and shop around for the best interest rates you can find. If after that you're still unsure which saving or investment schemes are best for you, it might be worth making an appointment with a financial advisor.

Instant or Easy Access accounts – open with as little as £1, access money easily, low and variable interest rates

Notice accounts – open with a few hundred pounds, need 30–120 days' notice to withdraw cash, variable but slightly higher interest rates

Fixed Rate accounts – minimum balance needed, and a fixed interest rate for a set period of time (if rates rise, you don't benefit, but if rates drop, your original rate is honoured)

Savings bonds – commit a set amount for a fixed term (say 1, 3 or 5 years), can't withdraw money in this time without penalties, low-risk savings option, guaranteed your money back plus interest

Cash Individual Savings Account (ISA)* – can only invest up to £3,000 per tax year, short-notice access (only a certain amount per day), but once you've invested £3,000 you can't put back in any money you take out, safe savings option and tax-free

Stocks and Shares ISA* – a long-term investment, usually required to invest an initial lump sum, then make regular payments, though can only invest up to £4,000 per tax year, involves stock market investment, so open to risk, although any gains are tax-free

> * You can only have two ISAs per tax year (one Cash up to £3,000 and one Stocks and Shares up to £4,000) or one Maxi ISA (must have a Stocks and Shares component but could have the full £7,000 as Stocks and Shares).

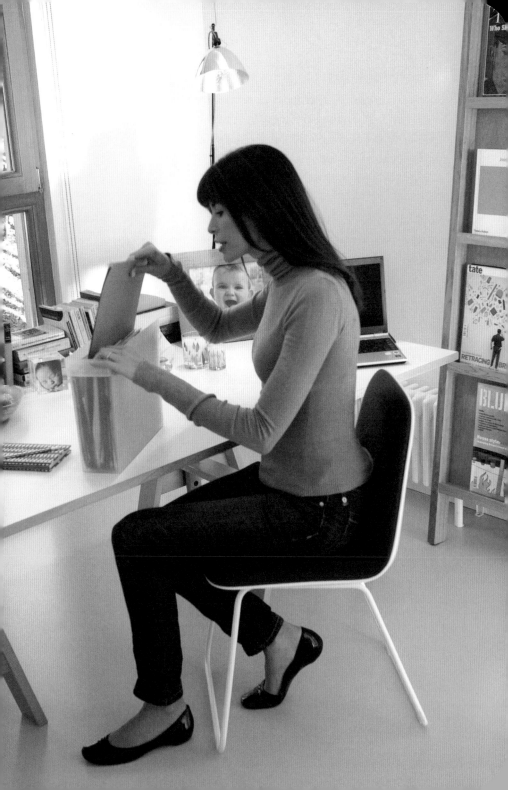

Your pension

No matter how far off it seems, it's never too early to start saving for retirement. If you haven't already done so, why not give yourself some peace of mind and look into setting up a pension fund? This involves paying a small part of your wages into a fund so that when you retire you'll receive regular payments based on your contributions. Fairly small changes in your budget planning now can make a big difference to your life in the future and also to how long you will need to continue working.

The earlier you start saving for your pension the better, because you earn interest from your savings. Even if you can only start with a small amount per month, it's still worth starting your pension, and you can always increase your payments as your earnings increase.

I've outlined a few types of pensions here, but with so many different schemes on offer, it's a good idea to seek professional advice.

Basic State Pension

- made up of National Insurance contributions taken from your wages by the government
- what you receive depends on how many years you've been contributing before state pension age (currently 65 for a man, and 60–65 for a woman)
- currrent pension is £87.30/week for a single person and £139.60 for a married couple
- although some costs of living reduce with age, others will not, so this is not a great deal to live off, meaning it's probably worth starting an additional pension

Company Pension

- set up by employers on behalf of their employees and promises a payment at retirement – a fixed proportion of an employee's earnings
- employers often make contributions on your behalf and you can make additional contributions direct from your wages if you choose
- find out if your company has a pension scheme, or if not, provides access to a group personal pension instead (you run your own personal pension plan but do so with other colleagues to reduce administration costs)

Personal Pension

- you can set this up if your employer doesn't offer a company pension or if you're self-employed
- you pay a regular amount and/or a lump sum to a pension provider, who invests the money on your behalf
- the most basic type is a stakeholder pension – with a minimum investment of £20 per month and no penalties for stopping contributions or transferring funds to another scheme
- charges are capped at 1.5 per cent per year and the amount of pension you get will depend on the size of your fund when you retire

Making a will

It was when I had my first child that the idea of creating a will first came to mind. Before that, I didn't worry about it, especially as I had no dependants. The fact is, kids or no kids, it's very important to have a will in place. Although it's unsettling to think about the prospect of your own death, if you have assets, such as a house, car, savings or jewellery, then you need a will. If you already have one, check that it's updated to reflect any major changes in your life.

Having a will, you could save your family complicated financial and legal battles if something unexpected happened to you. It also ensures that your property's distributed how you would like it to be, rather than according to the law. If you have a partner, bear in mind that if you don't have a will, they could end up with nothing.

Although it's possible to write your own will, it's advisable to use a solicitor to make sure the will is legal and valid. You may also need advice on more complicated topics such as inheritance tax.

Before visiting a solicitor, here are a few important things to consider.

- You must appoint one or two executors to be responsible for making sure your wishes are carried out and all trust documents are executed properly. Choose someone responsible whom you trust, and ask their permission and agreement before nominating them officially.
- To minimise your legal costs, do some research and understand as much of the process as possible before seeing a solicitor. The cost of writing up a will varies between solicitors and depending on how complicated your wishes are.
- Try contacting voluntary organisations that offer help with will writing. See my website for more details – www.lifestyle-essentials.com.
- Make a list of all your assets and decide who you would like to leave each item to (this is where the household inventory (see p.190) can come in handy).
- It's a very hard decision to face, but if you have children under eighteen you need to decide who to nominate as their legal guardian in the event of the death of yourself and their father.
- Consider any donations to particular charities.
- Once you have made a will, the solicitor normally keeps the original and sends you a copy. Keep it in a safe place and tell your executor, a close friend or a relative where it is.
- Review your will every five years or after any major change in your life, such as after giving birth to a child, moving house, a marriage, a divorce etc. Any change needs to be made by a 'codicil' (an addition, amendment or supplement to your existing will) or by making a new will.

- If your personal circumstances are complicated – if you run your own business, or have children from a previous relationship, for instance – you might need extra advice.

Your holiday

Travel is one of the many adventures of life, allowing us to experience different cultures, environments and climates. The world is an amazing and vast place, with so much to see and do – get out there and explore!

I've been very fortunate, through my various professions, to have been given the opportunity to travel to many wonderful places all over the world.

'My favourite thing is to go where I've never been'
Diane Arbus

Travelling can be exciting, adventurous and fulfilling but it can also be stressful and daunting, especially when you're visiting foreign and remote places. So, to travel well, you need to be organised. Though there are no guarantees when it comes to travel, the more organised you are, the more hassle-free your trip will be. The following tips should get you started.

Before you travel

- Make sure your passport is valid for the full duration of your trip
- Spend some time researching which countries and places you'd like to visit
- Search for the best deals for flights and hotels on the internet – go to www.lifestyle-essentials.com for some good links
- Check if you need a visa for any country you visit – it can take up to six weeks to process some visas

- Check whether you need any vaccinations – and if so, book an appointment with your doctor four to six weeks before you travel, as some require a series of injections or take time to become effective in your body
- Photocopy your passport so you don't have to carry the original around with you – this way you can leave it in a safe place
- Investigate the local currency and check what charges your bank makes on overseas payments and withdrawals. Some banks have low or no charges, so it might be worth investigating opening a special travel account. If you plan to order cash through your bank, do so well in advance of your trip as most don't hold every currency
- Purchase adequate travel insurance
- Check you have international roaming on your mobile, and if you're away for a while, consider getting a pay-as-you-go SIM when you reach your destination
- Create a checklist of all the things you need to do before travelling so you don't forget anything
- Leave your full itinerary, travel insurance details and a photocopy of your passport with someone at home, just in case of any emergencies

How to get there ... by air
- Search for the best deals and book flights as early as possible
- Offset the carbon cost of your trips through a carbon-offsetting company
- If possible, request specific seats when you book to ensure you're sitting with your travel companions, or to get an aisle or window seat. The seats at the emergency exits have the most leg room and are very popular so you'd need to request them early on
- Check in online – some airlines allow you to check in and select your seat before you get to the airport
- Request any special meals you require when you book

- If you hope to travel quite a bit, join the frequent flyer club of the airline you use to collect air miles towards your next holiday. Always give your membership number when booking your flight
- Drink plenty of water to prevent general dehydration as well as dryness in the nose, throat and eyes
- Drink alcohol and caffeine in moderation as they may cause dehydration and can disrupt sleep patterns
- Wear comfortable shoes and loose clothing as the body tends to swell while in the air
- Wear flight socks and try to move your legs and feet during a long-haul flight to maintain blood circulation and reduce the risk of deep-vein thrombosis (a blood clot)
- Be prepared – take snacks, reading material, a travel pillow, iPod, ear-plugs and anything else you need on the flight
- Be aware of check-in times when planning your journey to the airport and give yourself plenty of time in case of delays – avoid any last-minute panics and use any extra time to head to duty free!
- When booking more than one flight, be aware of the time needed to make a connecting flight, especially if you have to reclaim your luggage in between
- Check in advance hand luggage regulations at every airport you will fly from

How to get there ... by rail

- For making a booking and being prepared, follow the same advice as for flights
- Be aware of the best days and times to travel. Off-peak tickets are usually the cheapest and you are likely to have more room. Avoid commuter trains, where the fare will be higher and you might not get a seat
- Before you travel, check the appropriate websites for delays, maintenance works and bus replacement services, especially if you

need to be at your destination for a specific time. It's essential to do this if you are using the train to get to an airport
- Specify a seat, depending on your preference – if you hope to take in the view, request a window seat
- If you suffer from motion-sickness, make sure you sit in a seat facing the direction you're travelling in
- Investigate types of railcards available, especially if you plan to use the railway frequently, as you might be able to save money

How to get there ... by car
- Make sure your car is in safe working condition (see **Your car** on p.192) and check tyre pressure, oil, water and washer fluid levels before long trips
- If you're travelling a long distance, driving on your own, or use your car a lot, it's worthwhile investing in a breakdown service – so you can feel sure that you will be well looked after if you have any car problems
- Always plan your route, allow a suitable amount of journey time and never drive in a hurry. Make sure you take all the directions, appropriate maps and contact numbers you might need
- Take breaks when you need them, especially on a long journey, and never drive if you are overtired
- Pack plenty of snacks and water for your journey
- Remember to take your favourite music and audio books for entertainment along the way
- Take someone along for the ride – it's better for the environment and more fun!

Hotels
Although I stayed in lots of hotels throughout my modelling career, it wasn't until I met my husband and started travelling with him that I truly learnt the art of booking a hotel room. He is very particular

when it comes to choosing a hotel and room and he's taught me some invaluable tips.

For more travel checklists and tips visit www.lifestyle-essentials.com.

Hotel tips

- Before you make a booking, do your research. Find out as much as possible about the hotel and local area to make sure it has all the amenities you want and is in the right location. There's no point booking a lovely hotel for a beach holiday, only to find it's five miles from the coast! Similarly, if you are planning a busy, active holiday and you're using the hotel only as a base, you might not want a really plush hotel.
- If you have any special requirements, such as dietary restrictions, allergies, disabled access or internet availability, check that the hotel is suitable before confirming your reservation. Give as much information as necessary, ahead of time, to ensure your stay is as relaxing and trouble-free as possible.
- Let the hotel know if you have any room preferences, such as being away from lift shafts or busy streets if you're a light sleeper. There's no guarantee that you'll always get the ideal room, but you're improving your chances!
- When you check in, enquire about room upgrades. You have nothing to lose and it's worth doing, especially if you're checking in later in the day, because the hotel will then have a good idea of how many rooms are taken for the night.
- When you enter your room, check you're happy with it and that it will accommodate your needs. If you need to make a complaint or request, don't wait until later in the day or evening, as it may then be too late for them to change your room or organise the things you need.
- Be polite. The nicer you are to the staff at the hotel, the better service you're likely to receive. While tips are at your discretion,

I'd recommend tipping if you're looking for top-class service.

● If you're dissatisfied with any facilities or services during your stay, talk to the hotel manager immediately. A good hotel will try very hard to rectify the problem for you.

● Before checking out, ask for a copy of the bill to be sent to your room, especially if you have stayed for several days. This allows you to check in your own time that all charges are correct, rather than at the reception desk with others queuing impatiently behind you.

Your itinerary

Once you've chosen a destination, made your bookings and decided what you want to do on your trip, it's a good idea to create a travel itinerary with all the information you might need while on holiday. I keep a copy in my handbag and also email a copy to my Blackberry so I can easily find any information whenever I require it. Give copies to family and friends too, who might need to contact you while you are away.

Depending on your trip, you can include any relevant information you think would be useful to have in one place. As a guide, this is some of the main information you should include. You can download a proper template from www.lifestyle-essentials.com.

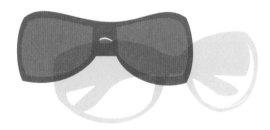

checklist

→ travel company details – contact name, number and email
→ dates of travel and timetables
→ destinations
→ flight details and check-in times
→ airline contact details
→ frequent flyer membership number
→ train/bus details
→ car rental agency contact details, reference number and membership number (if applicable)
→ insurance policy number and contact details
→ recovery policy number and contact details
→ hotel/accommodation address, contact number and reservation number
→ directions from airport/ station to hotel
→ places to visit/restaurants/ other ideas

What to pack

Whether you're off on a long holiday or a weekend break, packing can sometimes be a challenge. Most of us run around frantically on the day we're leaving, trying to remember everything we need before we head out the door – and that's why we're so stressed by the time we arrive at the airport. To prevent wasting a lot of time and paying any excess baggage fine, learn to be selective and organised about your packing. Think carefully about what you need and pack the minimum you require to look good and be prepared for any occasion. Make a checklist of what to pack, along with a last-minute list of what you need to grab just before you leave (eg. a charged mobile). If you set aside time for packing and check items off your list as you go, you'll feel much more calm and relaxed – trust me!

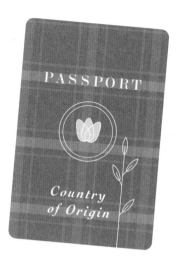

Some general tips

- Check weather forecasts a few days before you travel so you are prepared and can pack accordingly.
- For trips of one or two nights, only take hand luggage, if possible. It's easier to travel around without loads of luggage and you also save time at airports.
- Choose versatile items in neutral shades so they can be mixed and matched to create several outfits. Jeans are great because they can be dressed up or down for most occasions. To change the look of an outfit, pack small accessories such as a belt or necklace.
- Pick clothes that travel well and don't crease too much, as they can be worn out of the case.
- If you need to take delicate clothes, like silks, pack them with tissue paper to reduce creases.
- Try and pack clothes you can handwash – this way you can wear them again if necessary, or rewear in a different combination.

- Pack lightweight clothes if you can, depending on the weather. If you need a bulky sweater, try tying it around your waist rather than packing it. You can then place it in the overhead compartment on the plane.
- Shoes take up a lot of space so choose your most versatile pairs and try wearing the chunkiest or biggest ones (like boots or trainers) on the plane. Pack your shoes in individual fabric shoebags or even plastic bags so they don't dirty your clothing.
- Only pack the toiletries you will definitely use. Travel-size toiletries save you space, so bring back empty containers for your next trip.
- Check whether your hotel provides a hairdryer, as you may not need to pack yours.
- Remember to pack adaptor plugs for any electrical appliances.
- Always attach luggage tags with your contact details to all of your bags. As a double precaution against losing your luggage, write your contact details on a piece of paper and place it inside your bag or case, on top of the contents.

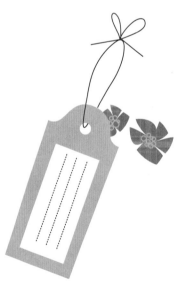

Packing checklists

Make sure you have a checklist for each different piece of luggage, including your main suitcase, your handbag, carry-on bag and toiletry bag. Travel templates for all of these are available on my website – www.lifestyle-essentials.com.

Before you fly, double check any weight, luggage and safety regulations for the airport and carrier. Many airports at the moment only allow you to take on a single piece of hand luggage – meaning you need to be able to fit your handbag inside your carry-on bag. You can probably only take liquids of up to 100 ml on board, and you must take these through security in a clear zip-lock plastic bag.

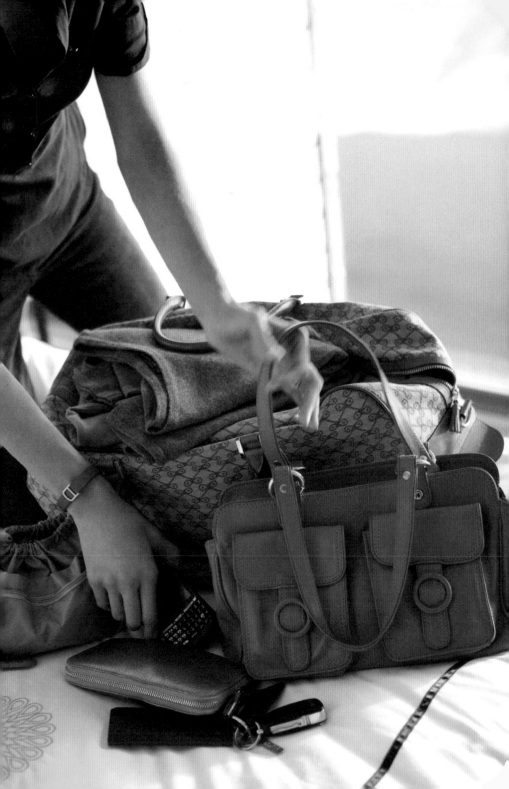

handbag

- [ ] passport/photo ID
- [ ] tickets
- [ ] frequent flyer card
- [ ] travel itinerary
- [ ] details/directions for accommodation
- [ ] map
- [ ] wallet
- [ ] foreign currency and small notes for tipping
- [ ] pen and notebook
- [ ] mobile/personal organiser
- [ ] iPod/mp3 player
- [ ] snacks/mints/chewing gum
- [ ] sunglasses
- [ ] handwipes/tissues

hand luggage

- [ ] books/magazines
- [ ] water bottle
- [ ] travel pillow
- [ ] eye mask/ear plugs
- [ ] camera/video camera
- [ ] laptop
- [ ] any leads/chargers/spare batteries
- [ ] international adaptor
- [ ] change of clothes/underwear
- [ ] present (for a host)
- [ ] toiletry bag

Arrive in style

To make sure you arrive at your destination looking your best, especially after a long-haul flight, I suggest the following tips.

- Wear comfortable yet stylish clothes (also remember – the more stylish your dress, the more chance you have of getting an upgrade)
- Make sure your clothes don't crease easily – whatever you do, don't wear linen!
- For really long-haul flights, and if you are wearing something businesslike or smart, consider bringing a change of clothes to put on after take-off, and then change back into your clothes before landing
- There is some very stylish casual wear at the moment – and even

tracksuits can look stylish these days. But if you do choose to wear a tracksuit, make sure the fabrics are good quality and that you're completely colour-coordinated
- Bring some make-up remover, cleanser and moisturiser so you can remove your make-up and reapply just before landing
- Bring a small hairbrush and hair band so you can tie your hair back if your hair isn't doing what you want it to do
- Try and get some sleep, so you arrive refreshed
- Bring a pair of large and fabulous sunglasses – hides a million sins!

Avoiding jetlag

After years of modelling when I had to travel to just about every time zone, I've certainly had my fair share of jetlag to contend with. It's doubly tiring because, in addition to usually not sleeping very well on the flight, jetlag disrupts sleep patterns and causes temporary insomnia while you adjust to the new time zone. While this generally takes about two to four days, there are a few things you can do to try and ease the period of adjustment and reduce the side effects of jet lag.

- Avoid drinking too much alcohol or caffeine, as it makes you dehydrated, and drink lots of water
- Try to eat before you get on the plane – you can choose healthier food. Or check if the airline offers low-calorie meal options before you fly
- Stretch regularly and take walks to stimulate your circulation
- Change your watch to the time of your destination as soon as the flight takes off
- If possible, slowly adjust your sleep schedule to be more in line with that of your destination a few days before you travel
- Try and get some sleep on the plane if you are flying during the night time of your destination
- Once you arrive, try and stay awake until it's bedtime rather than taking a nap

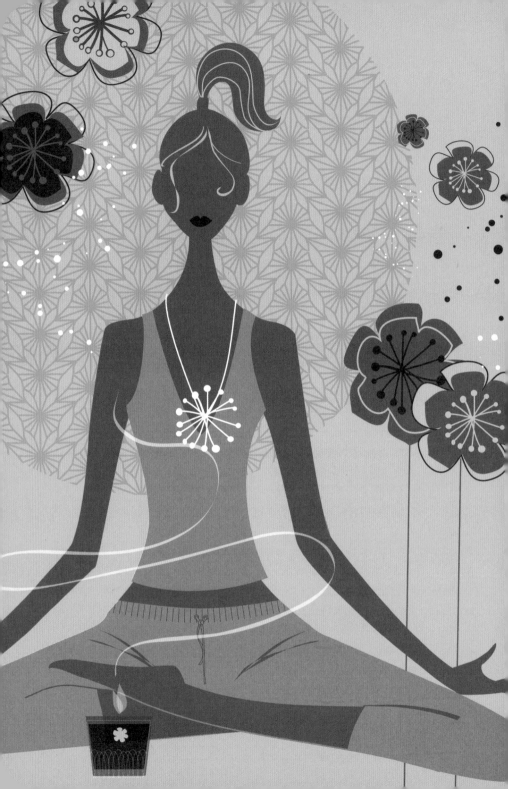

the 8 balanced you

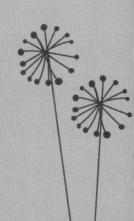

We've now looked at developing several parts of the essential you in the previous chapters – but the greatest fulfilment in life comes from protecting your own time and energy and finding a balance between them all. With so much to think about and so many ideas to pursue, it's easier said than done to fit everything in! Juggling all the things that require your attention – including your home, career, family, relationships and friends – alongside your own personal needs is going to be difficult. It's easy to feel guilty, frustrated and worn out while doing so, and there's sure to be a certain amount of trial-and-error as you learn what works and what doesn't.

In the end though, reaching some kind of balance is all-important. Making sure you're content with the way you live your life both within your home and outside it – with enough time for your friends, family and other pursuits – will help you to be more relaxed and generally happier. And surely, in the end, this is what all of us want ...

Dealing with stress

We've already talked about the serious effects of stress upon your body and health in **The Healthy You**. Now it's time to look in more detail at what you can do to understand and minimise the stress in your life. Perhaps the biggest cause of stress is our perception of losing control. When this happens, stress manifests itself in negative thoughts, anxieties and anger, which inevitably feeds back into our stress in one big vicious circle!

If you're feeling stressed out and need to address the balance in your life, think about how to implement the following pointers.

Prioritise

Take a look at the important parts of your life and put them in order of priority. Assess how much time you devote to each, which you want to give more time to, and which you can afford to give less time to. What is most important to you?

Plan and organise

Establish what needs to be done and when. Produce a schedule and stick to it, staying focused on the task at hand. By organising your time efficiently you can relieve some of the pressure – and both everyday tasks and long-term projects become more bearable.

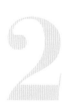

Delegate

Accept that no matter how organised, focused and driven you are, you will not be able to do everything. There just isn't enough time in the day, so learn to delegate and trust others to help you with certain jobs and tasks, especially your least favourite ones!

Don't be afraid to reach out to others and ask
for help when you need it; it might free up some
of your time to enjoy the other things in life.

Learn to say 'no'

Taking on too much and having an unrealistic
expectation of yourself will exhaust you and
ultimately lead to stress, unhappiness and failure.
By prioritising and delegating, as above, you can
learn to say 'no' to certain actions that are not
as urgent or as vital as others.

Allocate time to others

It is important to allocate time to the people who
are important in your life, such as your family and
friends. It is all too easy to get bogged down with
tasks that prevent you spending time with the
people who matter the most. If you're stressed,
share your thoughts with those closest to you – they
can offer help. They offer support, encouragement
and bring joy to your life, so don't take them for
granted, and make sure you offer them the
same support.

Create 'me' time

I must admit, I often struggle to set aside and enjoy
some 'me' time – it can be hard to relax and do
exactly what you want, without feeling guilty. But
it's important to try, because if you're not relaxed
and happy, you certainly won't make anyone else
happy, and you won't be as productive either.

Be aware of your own needs and set aside time to relax and unwind. Give yourself a treat and pamper yourself occasionally. It can be very therapeutic and will help keep the positive outlook on life you need to face the day-to-day challenges.

Try a little retail therapy or book yourself in for a beauty treatment; go out for the day or visit a friend you haven't seen for a while. You don't even have to spend money if you don't want to; you could get up late, have breakfast in bed and just take it easy all day, if you so wish!

tips

→ Exercise regularly
→ Eat a healthy, balanced diet and never skip meals
→ Stay away from alcohol and drugs – neither of these will help in the long run
→ Learn to control your breathing – maybe try yoga
→ Listen to calming music or relaxation tapes
→ Get away – take a break from the situation, whether for a few minutes or an actual holiday
→ Try stress-management techniques such as aromatherapy or reflexology
→ If you feel you can't keep stress levels under control on your own, never be embarrassed – seek professional advice

Stress at work

Work is a major source of stress at one time or another for most of us. Unfortunately, most of us do have to work, but what we don't have to do is let work and the associated stress rule our lives – you only live once!

If you're having a particularly stressful time at work, go to my website, where you can find some useful links to help you deal with your anxiety. In the meantime, here are some general tips for busting stress at work.

Exercise – Do some cardio exercises at the start of your day. During the day, get up and stretch at your desk or take a short brisk walk. Rather than phoning someone on a different floor – go upstairs to see them. Moving away from your desk really helps keep your energy up.

Drink lots of water – Heating and air-conditioning can really take their toll, so try to keep a large bottle of water on your desk to remind yourself to drink. Try to finish it daily so you don't get dehydrated.

Eat – Keep healthy energy-lifting snacks in your desk. Nuts and raisins are great, and so is fruit. I'd be lying if I didn't admit to my afternoon biscuit break at teatime (go on – treat yourself to a choccie biccie, just beware of having too much sugar throughout the day, as it can make your blood sugar drop).

Take a break – Taking short breaks can actually make you more productive over the course of the day. Make yourself a cuppa, share a joke with a colleague or step outside for a breath of fresh air.

Reconsider – If no matter what you do, you're always feeling stressed out by your job, then it's time to consider whether this is the right job for you and if it's worth it.

Working from home

Many employers these days are becoming more flexible about working part- or full-time from your home, while many people choose to be self-employed. Working from home can definitely give you a more flexible lifestyle, but it can also be tricky – it has both benefits and downfalls.

I often work from home and I know from personal experience that if your house is always full of kids and people, it's easy to be lured away from the task at hand. Setting clear boundaries between 'work time' and 'home time' can be problematic. On the other hand, not having to commute, and being at arm's length from your kids when they need you, is a joy.

If you've chosen to work from home, one thing's for sure: you need to be disciplined and self-motivated. Whether you already work from home, or are thinking about doing so, here are some tips that have helped me to juggle work at home successfully.

Choose something of interest

This is easier said than done, but if possible try and do something that you enjoy doing; this will keep up your interest and enthusiasm in your work.

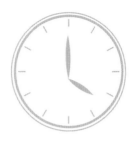

Create a workspace

Work from a specific workspace – designate an area where all you do is work and where you will start and end your day. Have the right equipment and systems to work with – an appropriate chair, desk, computer and filing system.

Define your hours

Be disciplined about the hours you work – they can easily get blurred when working from home and you can find yourself working either too much or too little. Create a schedule for yourself, including clear breaks, and follow it strictly. When your day has ended, shut your computer down so you're not tempted to fire off one more quick email.

Take time off

To avoid burn-out, take holiday time and sick days, just like you would if you were in an office. Taking a break and totally switching off from work allows you to recharge your batteries, leading to renewed enthusiasm and vigour, and greater productivity.

Constant input

Working from home can feel isolated, as you often lack external stimuli and influences. To keep you on the pulse within your field, study new skills or techniques, subscribe to industry publications and attend networking events.

Eliminate distractions

Remove and avoid any distractions – don't keep your television on when working, and if you have children, make sure their play area is at a distance.

Set boundaries

Friends and family may fail to respect your working hours – make sure you remind them that just because you're at home, it doesn't mean you're always available.

Balancing work and family

Time is always the key issue when juggling work and family. To manage both in harmony, you need to make a special effort to prioritise and get organised.

- Create a family calendar and hang it on the fridge so everyone can see it and add events.
- Make a list of things you need to do each week and prioritise them.
- Delegate – create schedules and routines for each family member and add to the fridge. Have certain days for laundry, cleaning, bill-paying and food shopping.
- Plan family meals ahead of time and buy food and household supplies in bulk.
- Get outside help if you can afford it. Your time's valuable, so free some of it up to enjoy with your family.
- Do at least one fun weekly family activity together – have a games or movie night on a Saturday, or spend Sunday afternoon in the park together. Put an activity in the diary each week and stick to it.
- Turn off the TV at dinner and talk.
- Have back-up plans and keep important numbers handy – especially of friends and family who can help you out with childcare if you need it.

When you've got kids, you always need to be prepared for emergencies.

- Stop being guilty! There's no right or wrong – working or stay-at-home. Both are as good as the other, as you are being the most loving and supportive parent you can be.
- Take care of you – you can't make anyone happy if you're not happy.

Download templates for lists, calendars, and menu planners from www.lifestyle-essentials.com.

Live in the moment ...

One of my favourite things to do when I wake is take in and feel that very moment. I am at my most relaxed.

I do a full body scan and visualise and feel everything around me, right from my head to my toes. I take a deep breath and feel how wonderful the sheets feel, how warm and cosy the duvet is, how soft my pillow is, how my body feels – if there are any aches and pains I should be concerned with – then do a great big stretch before I drag myself out of bed. It's a great way to start your day!

Spoil yourself

If life is a journey, why shouldn't it be filled with little treats along the way? We all need a little TLC sometimes, and who better to give it to you than yourself?

Spoiling yourself every now and then is a wonderful feeling and if you ask me, it's darn healthy too! With the busy stress-filled lives that so many of us lead, a bit of a pampering is wonderfully therapeutic and should be viewed as a method of survival, pure and simple.

If you're working hard and rushing through each day, then you owe it to yourself to claim back a little time for yourself, so go for it! Your mind and body will thank you.

Pamper tips

Weekend therapy – Take a weekend retreat. Book a holiday in the sun, or go and stay with friends you haven't seen for ages.

Retail therapy – Buy yourself a present. Try a new outfit, pair of shoes, piece of jewellery, new bath oil, a luxurious body cream or some heavenly perfume.

Edible therapy – Indulge yourself with a yummy treat. Try some chocolates, a bag full of pick-and-mix sweets, some caviar or champagne (or both together), a dinner out with friends, or pick a special bottle of wine.

Relaxation therapy – Dim the lights, play soft music, light scented candles and lie down and soak it all in. Try meditating. Or equally relaxing – get up late, have breakfast in bed, and if you feel like it, stay in your pyjamas all day!

Spa/beauty therapy – book yourself a massage, facial, manicure or pedicure – or the whole lot! Take a hot bubble bath at home with aromatherapy oils. Try creating your own spa at home.

Your home spa

Creating a soothing and relaxing atmosphere for yourself is every girl's prerogative. My two favourite rooms in my house are my kitchen and my bathroom – my kitchen because I love to cook and eat, and my bathroom because it's my pampering retreat.

When you're feeling the urge to escape, head towards the bathroom and prepare to treat yourself with a home spa.

1   Light the candles and, if you can, dim the lights (if not, just use lots of candles and keep the lights off)
2   Put on some relaxing music – soft nature sounds are perfect
3   Change into your soft robe and slippers. Tie your hair back and cleanse your face and apply a mask

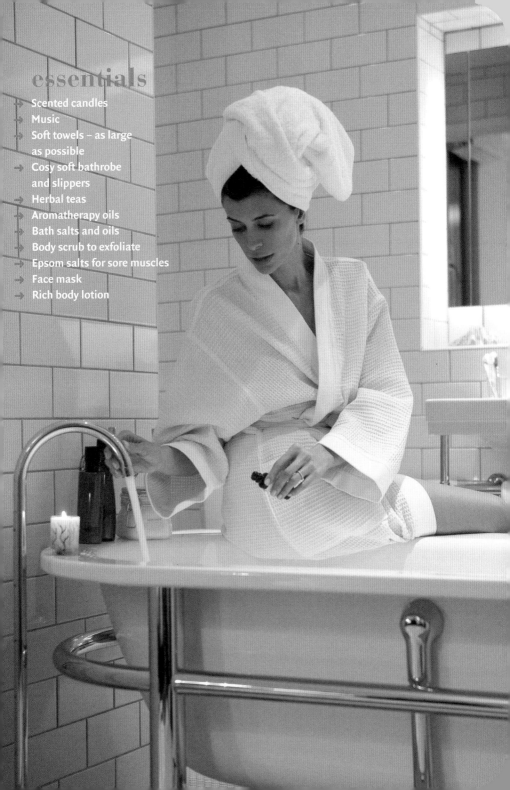

essentials

- Scented candles
- Music
- Soft towels – as large as possible
- Cosy soft bathrobe and slippers
- Herbal teas
- Aromatherapy oils
- Bath salts and oils
- Body scrub to exfoliate
- Epsom salts for sore muscles
- Face mask
- Rich body lotion

4 Draw a hot bath and add some bath salts or aromatherapy oil
5 Make yourself a mug of caffeine-free herbal tea
6 Get into your bath, close your eyes and relax ...

Singledom

I have to say, I love my husband, my married life and my young family and wouldn't change them for the world, but I also reflect on the joy and fun of being single. More than anything – because of my independent nature – I miss the spontaneity of doing things whenever you want to do them.

It doesn't matter whether you've never been in a long-term relationship or whether you've recently ended one – being single is a time when you have a whole lot of freedom, and can change your life as you see fit without impacting upon anyone else.

If you're newly single and grieving the end of a relationship, then it's without a doubt a painful period in your life. But the old saying holds true – time is the ultimate healer. I truly believe that in nearly all cases, people look back with hindsight and realise that a break-up was for the best – if they're not screaming 'What was I thinking?!'.

My mum used to say, 'What doesn't kill you, makes you stronger!', and I couldn't agree with her more – we grow from adversity, and hopefully become all the wiser and stronger for it.

If you've been actively looking for someone, then it might take some reflection to work out if there's anything holding you back from entering a committed relationship. Everything that we've talked about through this book – your manner, body language, energy, appearance, how you balance your time between work and play, your openness to meeting new people and experiencing new adventures – all of this makes up who you are and is ultimately what makes you attractive to someone else.

Or you may be content at the present time just as you are – to revel in your freedom, forge ahead with your own plans and adventures and make the most of being on your own! In which case, all power to you – keep doing whatever you're doing!

Whichever of these it is, make the most of the opportunities presented by singledom – it's likely they won't last for ever. The most important thing when you're single is that you feel happy with yourself – if you're not content, then it's time to look at what you'd like to change and which areas of your life you'd like to be more in balance.

Enjoy single life

Be happy with yourself – It's far better to be on your own than in a bad relationship which damages your self-esteem.

Channel your energy and focus – Being single allows you to arrange your time as you like, and put some extra effort into your work, a side project or hobby.

Stay social and active – Join clubs or workshops, or take a class in something entirely new. As you stimulate your mind and body, you expand yourself as a person – and feel happy in yourself.

Pamper yourself – Have massages as often as you can, or a wonderful spa treatment, or buy yourself some flowers.

Strive for financial independence – Make sure you won't compromise yourself in an unhappy relationship.

Nurture and expand your friends – Great friends will always be in your life, whether you're single or in a relationship. Make an effort to expand your circle of friends too – especially if you're trying to meet someone new.

Always live in the present moment – Be open and positive about where you are in your life. As soon as you stop fretting, worrying or focusing on being single, you'll be amazed how your energy changes and lifts. Not surprisingly, it's when you're happiest with yourself that you become more attractive and inviting to someone else.

Make sure they're worth it – If you've started seeing someone new, make sure they're worth giving up all the pros of being single for! Only stay in a mutually supportive relationship – you should be getting as much energy out of it as you're putting in.

Coupledom

A great relationship is one of the most wonderful and rewarding things you can have in your life. However, even the best relationships need constant effort, compromise and work from both sides. Two of the most important skills that help build and maintain a truly equal relationship are listening and talking. Communication is key to keep your relationships in balance, and if you can keep lines of communication open throughout any tense periods or disagreements, you can overcome almost any problem together.

10 steps to coupled bliss

1

Spend focused quality time together – Make sure you have enough time alone where you can be intimate and share thoughts, big and small. Make regular dates to go out just the two of you – to have a meal together, or do something both of you enjoy. Take a holiday together each year, without the kids, friends or any other distractions – make it about each other.

Be a good listener – This helps you understand your partner.

2

3 **Share your hopes, dreams and feelings** – Your partner will love to hear what the future may hold for you both – your togetherness, your plans for adventures, your family life. You should also share your feelings – both good and bad. Talk to each other not only when you're down, blue or afraid, but also when you're elated or happy about things in your life.

Establish boundaries – Be clear about your expectations, what you need and how you can help one another achieve this. **4**

5 **Confront issues** – This doesn't mean you should have a full-blown argument, but if you're not happy about a particular issue, then you need to voice it in order to resolve it. (Being Puerto Rican/Italian, I do think that letting off some steam occasionally can also be quite healthy for a relationship – and it leaves the making up to look forward to too!)

Agree to disagree – It's important to accept that differences of opinion are a normal part of relationships. You can't always agree with your partner – but it's important to realise that not all battles need a clear winner and a loser. Come up with suggestions for solving the problem or compromising, rather than placing blame. **6**

7 **Encourage and compliment your partner** – Acknowledge their achievements and efforts, especially in your life together. Everyone feels great after receiving a sincere compliment.

Empathise and be diplomatic – Put yourself in your partner's shoes and try to see things from their perspective. Don't make hasty statements without trying this first. **8**

9 **Share family plans and ideas** – Organise family holidays or outings and celebrations together.

Remember to laugh together – In too many relationships, the element of laughter fades after the early stages of romance. But laughing together is one of the best feelings in the world – so keep a sense of fun in your partnership.

10

Friendships

Besides my family, my friends mean more to me than anything else. They add richness to my life – they make me laugh, support me when I'm down, and guide and reassure me. But most of all, they make me feel blessed to have them in my life.

It says a lot about you if you have great friends – and whether you're single or in a relationship, friends should still be a vital part of your life. When you look back over the years, it isn't our accomplishments that have the most significance, but the people we connect with along the journey.

A true friendship can be a little like good health; you don't always realise the value of it until it's lost. So it's good to reflect from time to time on what your friendships mean to you, and check that you're keeping your friends in balance with the rest of your life. It can be difficult when you're juggling a busy lifestyle to give them the time that they deserve, but it's worth the effort – friendships do take nurturing and cultivating, but they give you back all of the energy that you put into them.

'When the character of a man is not clear to you, look at his friends.' *Japanese proverb*

Understanding friendships

All friendships are different and add diverse dynamics to your life. Most of us have several types of friends, and this is a positive thing – as long as we understand and accept these relationships for what they are.

True Friends – Cherish these friends and they will be with you forever. A true friend will be there for you whenever they think you need them. They are close enough to be honest with you, sometimes even telling you things you might not want to hear.

Long-distance friendships – Some of my dearest friends live far away, but this doesn't mean I value their friendship or think about them any less. If it's a true friendship, then the wonderful thing is you can grow separately without ever growing apart.

Fair-weather friends – I think we all have a few of these! These are the friends who appear when times are good, but can be a bit inconsistent and unreliable. Despite this, you might well enjoy their company from time to time. As long as you are aware and accepting of their shortcomings, then you can save yourself any disappointment with their friendship.

Making friends

- Trust your instincts when meeting new people – if something doesn't feel right, it generally isn't.
- Don't judge people before you meet them for yourself; some of my nearest and dearest are friends I might never have had if I'd judged them by the cover!
- Friendships need to be sincere – most people will guess if you are trying to be friends with them for the wrong reasons.
- Likewise, don't waste time on those who don't have your best interests at heart.
- Just go up and introduce yourself ... go on, what have you got to lose?

Nurturing friendships

Make time – Spend time with your friends. Do this by prioritising your personal time. Connecting with friends is essential to your enjoyment of life and inner well-being.

Appreciate them – Never take true friends for granted – and let them know they are special friends. Schedule a lunch or dinner date, send a handwritten 'just thinking about you' note, call for regular catch-up chats, remember their birthday, cheer them up when they're down, or go on a holiday together – make a real effort to be a consistent, reliable friend.

Be there – Friends love to see you during the good times, but they also need you during the bad. When a friend goes through a difficult or critical moment in life, they need your company. You don't have to have the perfect words – just your presence and your love will mean the world.

'The only way to have a friend is to be one.'
Ralph Waldo Emerson

Home sweet home

Your home is the centre of your life and has a huge impact on your sense of balance and well-being – it's where you find solace, comfort and security and where you can escape from the outside world. You want to feel safe and relaxed in your home, but sometimes the constant attention and work involved in running a home can disrupt the harmony. If your life at home is stressful then you will almost certainly pass the stress on to other aspects of your life.

For me, my home is my haven, where I can be my own person, do things the way I want to do them, and relax. Home is the place I would always rather be and I do all I can to keep it this way. This means paying attention to all the different elements that go into creating atmosphere – and that each room fits the purpose it's designed for. A bedroom should be a relaxing retreat, your kitchen needs to be practical and user-friendly, the living room welcoming and so on.

On top of that, my best general tips are keeping clutter to a minimum, having fresh flowers and scents around the home, and creating atmosphere with music and lighting. By making your home a special place it becomes somewhere where you love to bring friends, but most importantly, where you love to spend time yourself.

Get rid of clutter

I know I've been guilty in the past of being a complete pack rat – probably most of us have been at some point in our lives. But the truth is that clutter creates chaos, making it difficult to think or be productive – it can actually create more stress and even cause depression.

When we've got giant piles of 'stuff' everywhere, it becomes easy to put off doing anything about it, and within no time the clutter grows out of control. Every time you look at it, it tweaks your brain as a further something 'to be done'. So if stepping inside your front door after a day's work makes you cringe, it's time to do something about it. Get rid of the clutter and reap the benefits of living in a welcoming, clutter-free environment – you'll be that much more productive and relaxed.

- Start with one room at a time – begin by opening your curtains and windows to let in fresh air and light ... it's time for action.
- Start clearing out – place everything in the middle of the room and survey the clutter. Remember – you're trying to get rid of what you don't ever use.
- Throw out papers, catalogues and magazines which you know you've finished with – these are huge clutter culprits. Discard junk mail

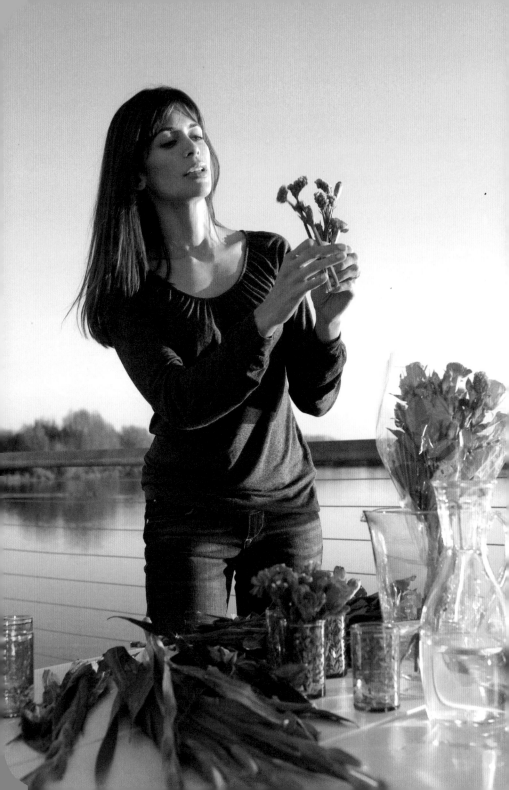

immediately and don't ever let it gather in your home.

- Create a filing system for important documents or articles and handle each item once – this goes for sorting your mail too. Divide into file, action, or pending.
- Donate or sell whatever you feel guilty about throwing out. Put all of these into black bin liners straight away, before you change your mind. Stick the bags for charity by the door or in the boot of your car ready to go, and post items to sell on eBay, or advertise locally.
- When you're left with everything you want to keep, assess your storage space and jot down how you can best use this.
- Use boxes and labels to store away things such as seasonal decorations, use small boxes to tidy up a chaotic drawer, shelves at the bottom of a hall closet to store shoes and outdoor gear, or roll-out drawers beneath your bed (pick ones with lids so stuff inside doesn't get dusty).

By this stage, things should be looking in pretty good shape, you should be feeling purged and good about yourself, and you can give yourself a pat on the back. After all this effort, make sure everyone in your household is responsible for their own clutter. If everyone actually tidies up after themselves, it's automatically easier to keep your place looking good. People are far more likely to clear up after themselves if there are only a couple of things out of place. Finally ... sit back and enjoy! You deserve your clutter-free haven!

Flowers

Flowers aren't just for giving to others – you should enjoy them too, so treat yourself whenever you can. Don't wait for a special occasion to have fresh flowers in your home, as they make can any day a little brighter. Put them somewhere eye-catching in your home to create a relaxing and welcoming atmosphere

I love using potted plants which flower seasonally. This way I can plant them in my garden when they've finished blooming and look forward to the blooms the following year. Orchids are great for dotting around the house – they look beautiful and elegant and last for ages.

When selecting cut flowers – go for flowers which are in season, as they tend to look better and will certainly cost you less. They offer richer colours, deeper fragrances and often last longer too.

Seasonal blooms

Summer – marguerites, campanulas, sweat peas, sunflowers, garden roses, cosmos, poppies, hydrangea, tuberose, agapanthus, carnations, delphiniums

Autumn – dahlias, achilleas, green lisianthuses, gladiolus, crocosmia, Chinese aster, foliage such as seeded greens, poppy pods, berries and star leaves

Winter – amaryllis, autumn hydrangea, early hyacinths, hollyberry

Spring – narcissus, daffodils, tulips, peonies, hyacinths, lilies of the valley, lilac, cherry blossom, viburnum opulus

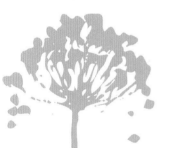

Flower tips

Whether you buy flowers or get them from your own garden, follow these tips so they look beautiful, stay fresh and bloom for longer.

- Select a vase that shows the bouquet off or complements their colours – consider bowls, pitchers and even tumblers as alternatives
- Cut the stems at an angle and strip any leaves or foliage that falls below the waterline
- When arranging flowers, try snipping some stems shorter, combining different colours and textures, and using foliage, buds, sprigs and other cuttings from the garden

- Fill the vase with fresh lukewarm water and add commercial flower food
- Every two days, change the water, add a sprinkling of flower food, and recut the stems if they've turned brown

Sweet smells

There's nothing more relaxing and welcoming than coming into a lovely-smelling home. The scent of your home says a lot about you – it reveals your thoughtfulness and attention to detail. A house that isn't cleaned often enough can give off a mouldy, damp or stale smell – definitely what you want to avoid!

One of my favourite ways to get a great-smelling house is from cooking, baking and roasting – what can beat the smell of a cake baking or a yummy roast in the oven? But an easier way is by using scented candles – which can be used for all occasions. You can use different scents in different locations to create an array of moods – from radiant romance to elegant formality to cosy comfort. Oil rings, which hide underneath lampshades by being placed on the bulbs, are also great for scenting your home, and pot pourri is lovely as long as it's the real thing (and not coloured wood shavings). Generally I give incense sticks a miss altogether as I think they tend to smell cheap and musky.

Uplifting and energising scents

These are great to use when getting ready to go out at night to lift your mood or when hosting a party. When your guests walk in, these scents will be a fresh breeze to welcome anyone. **Try: citrus scents, verbena, peppermint, rosemary, basil, lemongrass, pine and tea tree.**

Relaxing and stress-reducing scents

These are perfect for relaxing and winding down, for home spas or before you go to sleep. **Try: lavender, sandalwood, vanilla, amber, bergamot, patchouli, cedar wood, eucalyptus, ylang ylang and tuberose.**

Romantic scents

If you're trying to set the scene for romance, these scents should do the trick. **Try: jasmine, gardenia, sandalwood, rose, ylang ylang.**

Season-enhancing scents

Use certain scents to highlight the season. For example – choose spiced scents to create a cosy winter environment, or create summer by having a fresh citrus scent drifting through the air. **Try: pine, cinnamon, apple, berry, pumpkin spice, cedarwood, and wild currant for winter, and lemon, citrus, rosemary, mint, vanilla, and florals for summer.**

Music

Listen to music every day if you can, and have it as a regular feature of your home. I believe it feeds the soul, and as you can choose it to match whichever mood you wish – mellow and laid-back, or full of energy – it's much better than the background noise of unwatched TV chatter!

I put on my favourite tunes when I need inspiration, to keep me grooving when I'm cooking or doing housework, when I'm having a meal with my husband or friends, or when I just need to veg out and relax. By combining music with lighting, scents and flowers – you have everything you need to complete whatever atmosphere you desire.

You might have a favourite radio station where you listen to the latest releases, or you might have a favourite artist you always listen to – I know Kylie is always great for cleaning!

Having recently transferred all of my favourite CDs to my computer, I now have a few new addictions – making myself playlists and buying new songs from iTunes! I listen to my own compilations all the time now, whatever I'm doing, and use them when entertaining as well. For all of you closet DJs out there – this could be your moment to express yourself!

Lighting

One thing my husband and I definitely don't see eye to eye on is lighting. If he gets home before I do, you're guaranteed to need sunglasses to enter the house – every light in the place is blazing! Firstly, this is no good for the environment, and secondly, I find lower and more subtle lighting more warm and welcoming.

Lighting affects your comfort. It's incredibly important in both meeting practical needs and creating mood in a room – so it needs to be thought out carefully. To light a home with style, consider using several types of lighting in different areas of the room. Of course, you need to make sure that areas where you read, work or cook can be well lit when you need them to be, but otherwise, try to find a balance between not too bright and not too dim.

tips

→ Try installing dimmer switches so you can control the level of brightness easily

→ Use task lighting to light specific areas or objects instead of lighting an entire room

→ When lighting your kitchen, place light fixtures under cabinets and over work surfaces as well as using central fixtures

→ In the bathroom, make sure lighting is flattering – as well as central lighting, the mirror needs to be well lit to eliminate shadows under the eyes, nose, cheeks and chin

→ Candlelight creates a lovely soft and warm ambience – great for cosy nights in, relaxing bathtimes and entertaining

→ For the best, most flattering glow in your home – use a combination of soft lighting and candles

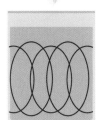

Candles last a lot longer if you place them in the freezer for at least three hours before burning.

Go green

As we all know, climate change is an increasingly serious problem that affects everyone on this planet. Originally, humans lived in perfect balance with their environment, but now the negative impacts of human behaviour are making themselves felt at an alarming rate. Even in the eighteen years I've lived in England I've observed obvious changes to the seasons – while worldwide, natural disasters seem to be striking faster than we can provide aid to the victims.

The time is past when we could say that climate change might only affect distant future generations. We have to worry about it and do something about it now, for ourselves, for our children, and for the Earth itself.

Human emissions of greenhouse gases, in particular of carbon dioxide, come through the burning of fossil fuels for energy and transport, and through clearing land of trees for agriculture. Levels of emissions are vast, far exceeding anything in human history, and need to be dramatically cut.

In the UK it's estimated that 40 per cent of carbon emissions come from business activity, 29 per cent from transport and 25 per cent from our homes, so it's definitely important that we all evaluate our lifestyles, take responsibility for the environment and see what each of us can personally do to help reduce emissions in our daily lives. Try to live a more balanced life by considering the environment in everything you do.

One of the best ways to help the environment is to look at how you can reduce your carbon footprint. A carbon footprint gives a measurement of the impact of human activity by looking at the amount of carbon dioxide you cause to be released.

→ Walk more
→ Buy organic
→ Recycle
→ Buy food in season
→ Don't print out
   documents unless
   you need to
→ Eat less meat
→ Take more trains
   instead of planes
→ Switch to renewable
   energy
→ Plant a tree!

Within my home I try to be as energy-efficient as possible – although when you live in a house always full of people, this can admittedly be tricky. At the moment, my husband and I are looking into switching the electricity and gas to renewable energy, but I know it's also the little things that do make a difference – from buying energy-efficient appliances to doing full loads of washing and using the coolest wash setting. Once you get into the habit of thinking about your daily actions, it really becomes second nature. It's up to all of us as individuals to do everything we can to collectively reduce the impact of our daily lives on the environment. So go on, what are you waiting for?

At home

These tips can help you save energy at home, which not only reduces emissions, but also your energy bills – as good for your bank balance as the environment!

Daily energy savers

All of these are ultra-easy and ultra-cheap ways of helping you save energy at home.

- Look for the Energy Saving Recommended logo when you buy appliances – they will be more energy-efficient than other products.
- Turn electrical appliances off rather than leaving them on stand-by.
- Use appliances efficiently – only run your washing machine or dishwasher when full (don't do small loads), and hang your clothes out to dry rather than using a tumble dryer.
- Wash clothes at 30 rather than 40 degrees – reducing your washing machine's electricity consumption by an average of 40 per cent.

- Choose detergents which work efficiently at lower temperatures, although it might be necessary to wash towels, sports gear and bedding at a higher temperature.
- Defrost your fridge and freezer on a regular basis.
- Use energy-saving bulbs in your home.
- Make sure your boiler system is efficient and in full working order.
- Review how you use your heating timers and thermostats – only have your heating running when you really need it. By putting on a jumper and reducing your thermostat by just 1 degree, you could save up to 10 per cent on your heating bill.
- Burn natural materials, such as wood.
- When doing DIY, look for wood products that show an FSC (Forest Stewardship Council) label or something similar – to show that the wood's been produced sustainably.

Daily water savers

The average person in the UK uses 135 litres of water a day – a mind-boggling amount, especially when you consider that most people don't even drink the 2 litres a day that they should! Here are some easy ways to help stop water wastage.

- Fix dripping taps straight away, to reduce water wastage.
- Consider installing a low-flush toilet or add a water displacement device to the cistern of your existing toilet – to reduce water wastage when flushing.
- Save the long, hot baths for when you really need to relax – a five-minute shower uses only a third of the water.
- Turn the tap off while you're brushing your teeth or washing up dishes – don't leave it running.
- Only boil as much water as you need in the kettle.
- If you have a garden, water it in the early morning or late evening – the water doesn't evaporate as quickly and your plants will feel the benefits too.

Long-term energy savers

If you want to get really serious about having an environmentally friendly home, then here are some alterations you can make. These can obviously cost quite a bit, but will really help reduce the level of emissions from your home.

- Reduce heat loss through your walls and roof by insulating your house – for instance, look into cavity wall insulation.
- Reduce heat loss through windows by installing double-glazing or by using draught-proofing products.
- Insulate your hot water tank.
- Consider using renewable energy options if possible, such as solar or wind power – most of the larger companies offer competitive quotes now, with discounts for switching.

For helpful links, visit my website – www.lifestyle-essentials.com.

Recycle and reuse

Recycling or reusing as much of your household waste as possible is a crucial step, because it means a reduction in both the need for landfill sites and in the energy and raw materials required to make new products.

Recycling doesn't just mean putting out your recycling box each week – there are a number of other ways to avoid being wasteful. My kids seem to grow out of their clothes quicker than I can blink – so I pass the clothes on to friends with children, or donate them to charity. Toy swaps are another great idea if you have kids – no more complaints about being bored!

Other ideas to get you started

- Nearly two-thirds of household rubbish can be recycled, so take a careful look at your waste and make sure you recycle everything that you can.
- Check to see if your council runs doorstep collections of paper, glass, plastic and sometimes even metal and organic waste, and make sure you use all services available.
- Find out from your council where you should take waste that they don't pick up – locate your nearest recycling centre and find out what they accept (they should take electrical appliances, wood and other waste).
- Sell clothes you don't want on eBay or swap with your friends – green is the new black!
- Give old clothes and linen to charity or a clothing bank so they can be reused.
- Don't throw away mobile phones – most local phone shops will recycle them.
- Cut down on excess packaging – where possible reuse carrier bags and invest in sturdy grocery bags.
- More than a third of household waste is organic, so if you have a garden, start a compost heap.
- If you don't have a garden, most councils also collect green waste – if they don't, ask them to recommend a suitable compost disposal method. Some authorities pass on compost to be used for soil improvement locally.
- If possible, buy products made from recycled goods, especially paper.
- In the garden, use a watering can instead of a hose to water your plants. Ideally, invest in a water butt to collect rainwater as well.

For more about going green, visit www.lifestyle-essentials.com.

Go organic

Why go organic?
1 Better for the environment
2 Fewer pesticides
3 No genetically engineered ingredients
4 Tastes better
5 Less intensive farming and more respect for soil structure and wildlife

It really is worthwhile eating organic whenever and wherever possible. Non-organic food can unfortunately be accompanied by a range of nasties that you really don't want to be putting into your system. To give you an idea, let's look at a few common foods to see why you should be choosing organic.

Milk – Scarily, antibiotics and hormones are routinely added to cows' feed and can find their way into milk.

Fruit – Choosing organic is especially important for fruit with edible skin, particularly berries – which grow close to the ground and get doused with a higher concentration of herbicides, fungicides and insecticides.

Lettuce/salads – Artificial fertilisers are used to grow lettuces. Choose whole organic lettuces rather than pre-washed bagged loose lettuce, as it's often been washed in chlorine.

Chicken – Buy organic and free range! Aside from the horrors of battery-farmed chickens, non-organic chicken also contains growth hormones and antibiotics.

Eggs – Levels of pesticides and antibiotics can be even higher in eggs than chicken.

Pork – Pork is one of the most intensively produced meats, which means it's most likely to be filled with antibiotics.

Beef – Organic cattle must be able to graze outside, meaning the meat contains more omega-3 oils and less saturated fats.

Shopping ethically

Today's consumer world is one of endless choice – yet we often don't even think about the choices we have. The power of the consumer in making buying choices shouldn't be underestimated, so here are a few tips on how you can put some thought into your next shopping trip.

- Always try to shop locally
- Buy seasonal food produce, and make it organic or free range wherever possible
- Avoid cheaply produced clothing from sweatshops, where there are often abusive labour practices
- Look out for organic clothing – it's becoming increasingly easy to find
- Buy Fairtrade
- Buy products you can recycle

Being charitable

Charity work is the elixir of my soul. Aside from monetary donations, these days I probably devote a third of my time to charitable causes – when it comes to charity I find it almost impossible to say no. I give my time in various ways – some of these include participating in charity fashion shows and working on committees, while I'm also a patron or ambassador for several charities that I endorse through the media.

The most important thing is to find a cause you feel passionate about. I remember reading an article about fourteen years ago, which uncovered the plight of the moon bears in China. The story was so horrific, I was crying before I could finish reading it. I immediately made contact with the charity (IFAW) to see what I could do to help, and have been a supporter and ambassador for their Animal Action Week ever since.

Once I had my first child, I soon added child welfare to my list of concerns. To me, animals and children represent innocence – they don't have the voices to clearly articulate their suffering, and they deserve our protection. Last year I went to Romania to see for myself the plight of institutionalised children. It was heart-wrenching to see so many children abandoned without being loved, touched, or even fed properly. This trip saw the birth of my charitable campaign Mothers4Children – which I hope will eventually turn global and be able to help fund smaller charities that are most effective in all areas of child welfare.

Visit the website at www.mothers4children.org.

Any kind of charitable giving you can manage – whatever the level or amount – will make a difference to someone else's life, so it's important to remember that contributing individually is worthwhile. There are many ways you can give to charity and you don't have to break the bank with all of them either.

Being charitable really comes down to thinking about other people, and giving something – whether it's money, time or support – that will in some way help them. To lead a truly well-balanced life means also spending time thinking about others and doing what you can to improve their lives. On a day-to-day basis, this could include very simple things, like helping an elderly person on the stairs, stopping to give directions to a confused-looking person with a map, or smiling at the person behind the counter in your local store and asking about their day.

When it comes to donating to charity, this is a very personal thing and you may be passionate about a particular cause. If so, find out how you can most usefully contribute to it. Always make sure the charity is registered so you're sure your donation is being used in the best way possible. Here are a few options to consider.

Donate used goods

Have a look around your house and collect anything you no longer use or need. Check that all items are in good condition and then take them along to a charity shop or to a local event raising money for charity – such as a jumble sale. Some charities are even willing to arrange pick-up collections. There may be some items that charities won't take, such as electrical equipment, so check with them beforehand.

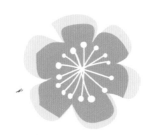

Donate your time

Visit charity websites and keep an eye out in your local paper to see if there are any events being run in your area that want volunteers. Just a few hours of your time can be a great help to others and hugely rewarding for yourself.

Organise an event

Look into organising a fundraising event for a particular charity you'd like to support. It could be anything from a coffee morning or car-boot sale, to a sporting event or a charity dinner dance. Explain a bit about the work of your chosen charity to anyone attending your event so they understand where their money is going.

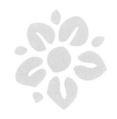

Giving money

There are several ways to do this, depending on how much and how often you want to give. Give a one-off gift or make regular donations by setting up a monthly or annual direct payment – contact your bank or the charity to find out the best way of doing this. Or you could set up a Charity Aid Foundation (CAF) account. This acts like a bank account for charitable giving, allowing you to donate easily to any registered charity you choose.

Gift Aid

Make a Gift Aid declaration with any donation. You just need to declare that you are a UK taxpayer and that you want the charity to receive back the tax paid on your donation from the Inland Revenue. Charities can send you a form to sign or will simply have a check-box for you to tick at the time of donation. There's no extra cost to you, while the charity receives extra funds.

Payroll giving

You can make a regular donation to a registered UK charity by using a direct deduction from your wage. The money is taken out of your pay before tax, so it's tax effective for you and again, the charity benefits, as they receive your donation plus the tax you would have paid on it. Ask your payroll or accounts department for more information.

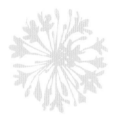

Legacies

Another way of giving to charity is to leave a designated amount in your will. You need to be specific about the charity or charities and the amount you want to donate. This is usually a way of giving a larger amount.

For more information on UK charities and ways of supporting them, head to my website for some useful links. Go to www.lifestyle-essentials.com.

The creative you

So many of us these days focus too hard on a single part of our lives, such as our work or family, and juggle this with all the mundane daily tasks that have to be done. But in order to have a balanced life and to feel good in your daily endeavours and routines, you also need to nurture your creative side. Being creative makes me feel great – so I indulge in it whenever I can.

Being creative means using imagination and originality in some way. Some of us are afraid to unleash our creativity, while others deny that it exists at all. However, all of us have a creative side – it's just individual expression, although it manifests itself in many different ways.

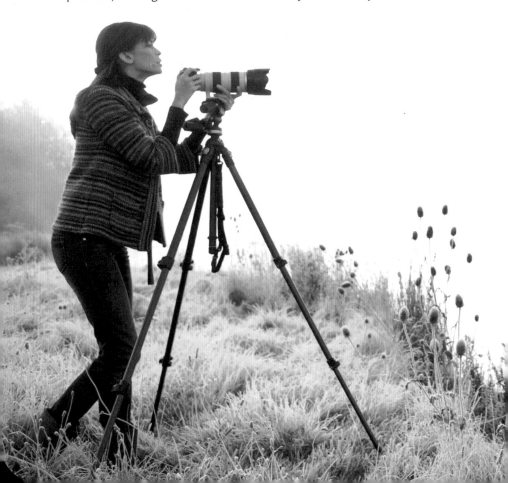

If you don't already have a creative outlet, then you need to find something that absorbs and inspires you and allows you to take a break from everything else that's going on in your life. There are countless ways to channel your creativity – so try out an evening class, join a club or group, or set aside the time to work alone on a particular creative project.

Here are just a few ideas, and there are many more, so you're sure to find something that suits you perfectly.

Inspirational ideas

- Creative writing – stories, plays, poetry, journal or travel diary
- Art – drawing, painting, sculpting, photography
- Music – instrumental or choral
- Dancing – any of a variety of styles
- Acting – an amateur dramatic group
- Cooking
- Gardening or flower arranging
- Martial arts
- Homeopathic or beauty skills – aromatherapy, massage or make-up artistry
- Crafts – pottery, knitting, sewing
- Photobooks and photo journals

Sometimes it can be difficult to get the creative juices flowing, so when I need creative stimulation, I try one of the following.

- Listen to or play music to evoke emotion and inspire creativity, or dance – interpret the music in your own personal way
- Read books and poetry to open your mind to different perceptions and thought processes
- Watch a thought-provoking or moving film
- Take a long walk to clear your head – I find parks, the countryside and beaches the best for this
- People watch – observing the individuality of others can be very inspiring
- Go to a museum, gallery or exhibition
- Attend the theatre or a concert

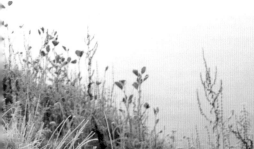

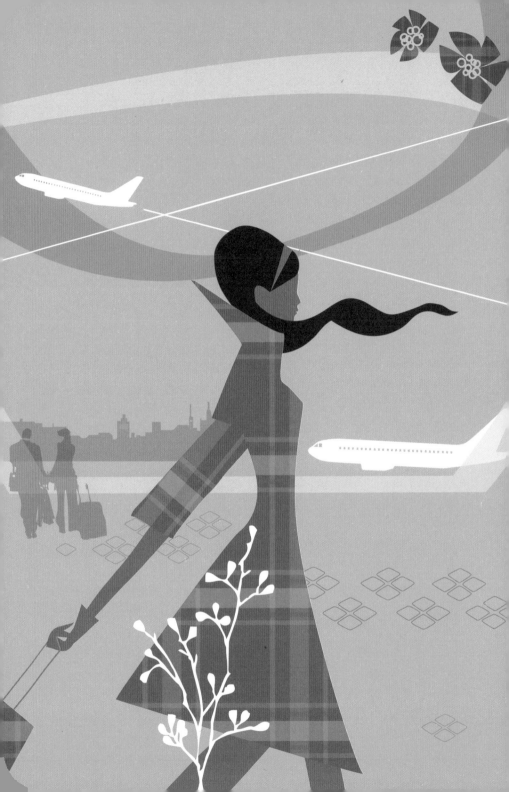

the aspirational you

9

Aspirational living is all about pursuing and living a rich and fulfilling life. It encompasses everything that we've discussed throughout this book – it's the effort that we put into each area of ourselves that can make our lives aspirational.

The aspirational you is what drives you to be everything you want to be – it's the you which gives you spirit and sets no boundaries. Your aspirations are what energise, excite and enthuse your soul, and reflect your appetite for life.

In all of the previous chapters you've been taking stock of your life and have assessed many of the factors that influence you and your lifestyle. You have identified, evaluated and learnt how to work on several important parts of your life to enable you get the most out of it.

After appraising your lifestyle, you may feel ready to achieve more. If you can channel your positive energy and use your determination and passion to look at new ideas and experiences, then nothing can hold you back. It's just a case of getting out there and pursuing your aspirations!

Aspire to be ...

Positive – Have hope, enthusiasm, optimism and vivacity. When you're positive, you have a higher sense of well-being and are more resourceful – you're better able to deal with whatever life throws at you and can go out and make things happen.

Generous and gracious – Be hospitable, open, unselfish, magnanimous and charitable at every opportunity.

Grateful – Acknowledge all the positive things in your life and also make sure you value yourself. Appreciate others too, and be respectful and appreciative of the life all around you.

Adventurous – Be open to new experiences, travel and pursue your passions.

Creative – Be innovative, inventive and creative. Use your imagination, be playful and continue to learn, dream and be inspired.

Focused – Be engaged, driven and organised. Take the initiative and apply yourself to reach your goals.

'There isn't a person
anywhere that isn't
capable of doing more
than he thinks he can.'
Henry Ford

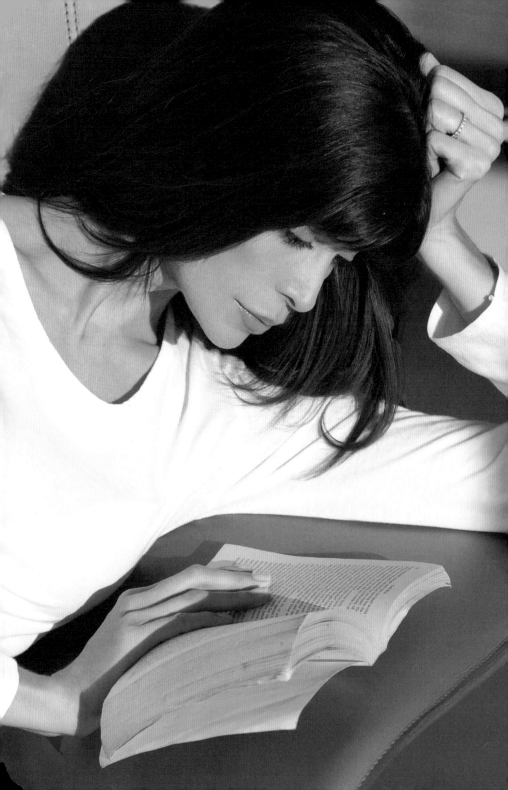

Broaden your horizons

When striving for success, it's incredibly important to develop and maintain a positive outlook on life, and convince yourself that you're capable of doing anything you put your mind to. We talked about the power of positive thinking in **The Essential You**. Use this positive outlook and inner confidence to broaden your horizons and cultivate new ways of keeping life interesting and inspiring.

> *'There are no limits to growth because there are no limits on the human capacity for intelligence, imagination and wonder.'*
> *Ronald Reagan*

In addition to self-confidence, your knowledge and awareness are helpful tools for giving you the drive and ambition to achieve more. Expanding your mind doesn't have to be a deep and heavy intellectual trip – it's more about being constantly inquisitive and aware of what's going on around you. Don't let your mind be lazy. Just as physical activity keeps your body strong, mental activity keeps your mind sharp and agile. An ex-boyfriend of mine used to say, 'You know Lisa, you've gotta have input to have output', and he encouraged me to soak up information and learn from people around me.

If it helps, make up a list of any subjects or experiences that interest you and encourage yourself to look into them one by one. And when you come across an interesting topic or subject during conversation that you know little about, make the time to investigate it further. A good grasp of general knowledge and current affairs topics not only stimulates your mind, it has the added bonus of making you more interesting company for others.

There are many ways to develop your general knowledge and keep up to date with new ideas. Here are a few of them ...

- Read a variety of books, newspapers and magazines
- Take an evening class or course
- Watch interesting and thought-provoking movies, documentaries and current affairs shows
- Use the internet as a research tool
- Experience new cultures through travel or studying a language
- Meet new people – show a sincere interest in and learn from their experiences

Embrace change

Creating a bigger and better life for yourself almost always involves change. Change can often be difficult – both to make and to adjust to. This means that change must come from within yourself, as it will only happen if you want it to happen.

You can rarely make a change if your heart's not in it. You need to have a passionate reason to change and a clear beneficial outcome – whether it's to increase your fitness to keep up with your kids, be organised to reduce your stress level, get out of a bad relationship to regain self-confidence, or stop smoking to improve your health. Once you grab hold of a strong reason and know why you want to change, then you're halfway there.

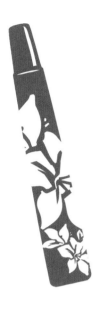

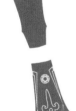

My essential journal

This is an exercise you can use to look at what changes you'd like to make. It really helps when you feel you're losing focus on where you want to be in your life. All you need to do is sit down with a pen and notebook and create a journal by trying to answer the following questions as best you can.

- What do I want more abundantly in my life?
- What do I want more of in my life?
- What do I feel is missing from my life that would bring me fulfilment?
- What do I already have that I am grateful for?
- What did I love to do as a child, but have given up?
- What are my strengths and talents?
- What dreams have I allowed to fade away?
- What would I do, if I had the choice to do anything?
- If this were do-able and I pursued it, what actions would I need to take?
- What am I willing to do and not willing to do in order to facilitate this?
- What would I be willing to sacrifice in order to accomplish my goal?

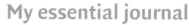

'They always say time changes things, but you actually have to change them yourself.' *Andy Warhol*

Achieving your goals

Throughout Lifestyle Essentials, we've talked a lot about setting goals, however big or small they are. And we've just talked about the need to embrace change. Knowing why you want to change and having a definite purpose is the key to your success in accomplishing a goal. How can you go somewhere if you don't know where you want to go? If you have purpose, you have direction. And with direction, you won't waste time doing things that prevent you from getting to where you want to be.

You can develop all the different elements of your life by setting, pursuing and achieving goals – whether your goal is to stick to a diet, organise an event, save for a holiday, up your career, be creative, or take on any new challenge.

When setting yourself goals, make sure they're realistic and allocate a suitable timescale for achieving them. Keep track of your goals by dividing them into long-term and short-term categories. I make a list of both and then prioritise them so I can deal with the most important ones first. For each long-term goal, I add mini goals, and then I often break these down further into tasks. Tasks are less daunting and you can cross each one off your list as you accomplish it. This feels great because you can actually see progress happening, making you realise that every little step takes you closer to achieving your ultimate goal.

'The key to realizing a dream is to focus not on success but significance – and then even the small steps and little victories along your path will take on greater meaning.'

Oprah Winfrey

By setting goals, you should be able to use your time more productively and efficiently. Just be willing to take some risks and don't expect too much too soon. If you believe in yourself and stay focused, you'll work harder to achieve your goals and will be more likely to succeed. As you achieve your goals, your self-confidence will increase too, motivating you to aim even higher.

Remember ...

It's very important to cultivate all areas that shape your life, but you also need to find a balance between them that allows you to get the most out of life and leaves you feeling content and fulfilled.

One thing you must always remember is that nobody is perfect and we all have our bad days – no matter how positive we are. Life is a constant rollercoaster of emotions and challenges, and by developing our self-awareness, we are equipping ourselves with the tools and knowledge to overcome any obstacles in our path. If you ever seem to be stuck in a rut, remember to take each day as it comes, as a moment that you can deal with and move on from.

Accepting and nurturing who you are and what you have is an important element of personal development. By understanding the components of the essential you and finding the balance between them, you can set and achieve goals, live life to the full and be successful in whatever path you choose to take.

Aspire to be the best you and live the best life you can – a life that's ultimately balanced, happy and fulfilled!

Be thankful

This book has talked a lot about how we should aspire to improve our lives, but it's also immensely important to appreciate what we already have. Gratitude can give you incredible strength and energy – so you should harness this force into your everyday life.

Life is a gift – our family and friends, the creative arts, the natural world around us, the sunshine and the air we breathe. We also need to appreciate our inner selves, our health and our bodies and how blessed we are – by our capacity to love and be loved, to feel, understand and show emotion, and even to create new life!

Try looking at things with the eyes of a child and see the world as new, wonderful and exciting. I'm in complete awe of our universe and grateful for every day that I'm a part of it ...

'To live is the rarest thing in the world. Most people exist, that is all.'
Oscar Wilde

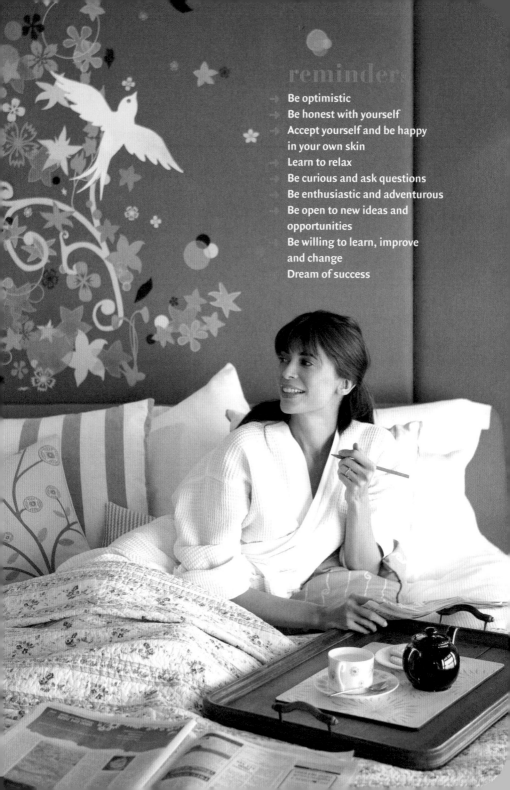

reminders

- Be optimistic
- Be honest with yourself
- Accept yourself and be happy in your own skin
- Learn to relax
- Be curious and ask questions
- Be enthusiastic and adventurous
- Be open to new ideas and opportunities
- Be willing to learn, improve and change
- Dream of success

Index

Acknowledgements

The end result of this book has come a rather long way since its conception. What started out as my own little 'Household Protocol' on a simple PowerPoint program (created mainly for my own sanity) soon evolved into a 'Pregnancy Organiser' (again – for my own sanity!) which was a result of my first pregnancy. You may have guessed by now – I like trying to keep things organised! When Peter Pugh at Icon Books agreed that I might be on to something, I was thrilled at being given the opportunity to properly pen my thoughts and ideas on all that encompasses modern lifestyles.

After handing in what could arguably be considered a book the size of a Yellow Pages phone book (or four more of these books!), I have a few people to thank for helping me create something I am really thrilled with and excited about.

Thank you, everyone at Icon Books who played a part in the creation of this book: Peter Pugh for saying 'Let's do it' and believing in me, Simon Flynn for overseeing and guiding me throughout the various stages of this project with discerning forethought, and Lucy Leonhardt, Tansy Hiner and Sarah Higgins who all helped to tie it together!

Thank you, Allan and Emma from Smith & Gilmour for their part in making this book look as beautiful and polished as it does, and for the enchanting and individual illustrations created by Barbara Spoettel, which embellish it so wonderfully.

Thanks to Colman Getty PR, for all of your efforts involving press and media – Mark Hutchinson, Vanessa Hammond, but in particular, Katie Morrison for your enthusiasm, guidance and 'getting my vision' for this project!

Partnering this book is the very exciting website www.lifestyle-essentials.com. I'd like to thank the team at Clevertech, particularly Colin Collino and Andy Derrick, for their technical genius and input in helping me develop and bring this side of the project to life.

To my nearest and dearest ...

A SUPER BIG thank you to my right-hand girl – Cristina Trica – who has seen every stage of every project I get inspired by, obsessed by and even possessed by! Thank you for all of your endless time, effort and involvement, your help with the research and your caring dedication to my vision(s!).

A big thank you to Trevor Leighton for the beautiful photos throughout the book and on the cover, for always being up for a 'Lisa B project' and a super Gemini twin – you are always so generous with your time, spirit and Northern humour – and you take a pretty darn great photo too! Long may you take my photo!

Thank you to Tara Smith – my Make-up and Hair Styling Guru – for working your magic and always giving so generously of your time and spirit.

Thanks to all of my lovely, yummy and individual friends (including the crazy ones!), and my family who all in some way are a part of or have influenced this book! Xxxxx!

And last, but certainly not least! My BIGGEST heartfelt thank you is to my husband Anton, your own enthusiasm and energy for life has fed the last five-and-a-half years of my life! I have you to thank for achieving this book – you constantly inspire me and because of you, I have my beautiful children who seem to innately put so much into perspective. Thank you for your support, encouragement and guidance, but most of all, your PATIENCE while writing this book ... Big love ... x